George Bournich

LaFreniere
Body Techniques

A Therapeutic Approach
by Physical Therapy

Joan G. LaFreniere, Ph.T.

Director
Physical Therapy Treatment Center
New York, New York

Distributed by
YEAR BOOK MEDICAL PUBLISHERS • INC.
35 EAST WACKER DRIVE, CHICAGO

▐▐ MASSON Publishing USA, Inc.
New York • Paris • Barcelona • Milan • Mexico City • Rio de Janeiro

Library of Congress Cataloging in Publication Data
LaFreniere, Joan G.
  LaFreniere body techniques.

  Bibliography: p.
  Includes index.
  1. Physical therapy. I. Title. [DNLM: 1. Physical
therapy. WB 460 L169L]
RM700.L24 1984   615.8'2   83-25622
ISBN 0-89352-205-8

Copyright © 1984 by Masson Publishing USA, Inc.

ISBN 0-89352-205-8

Library of Congress Catalog Card Number: 83-25622

Printed in the United States of America

Preface

Body Techniques is a new and unique system of health care through physical therapy. Therapist and patient alike will benefit from its use because of its varied applications to short-term treatment of pain and also to longer-term treatment by corrective and preventive measures. It is a system of evaluation, differential diagnosis, treatment, and/or preventive medicine, depending on which Techniques are emphasized by the therapist. Although the Techniques are easy to perform, all of the therapist's knowledge, skill, and experience are required to interpret the results and to decide on the proper application of its Techniques for maximum patient benefit.

The five areas of treatment included in Body Techniques are relaxation, joint and soft tissue mobilization, acupressure, spray and stretch techniques, and postural adjustments, which are further augmented by modalities and therapeutic exercise. These Techniques are presented in a manner designed to assist the therapist in applying them for both evaluation and treatment. Therefore, this book stresses manual physical therapy with *applications* and *interpretation* rather than basic skills and anatomical details. Its purpose is not to teach individual techniques, but rather to give instruction in the effective application of manual physical therapy methods learned in the conventional manner. This is a clinical "how-to" book that presents evaluation and treatment in a "laying on of hands" environment. It will train a therapist to use his or her hands as sensing organs to pick up valuable information necessary to identify precise etiologies of pain and areas of mechanical imbalance. This information will also help to decide the emphasis of future treatment protocol on an individual basis for optimum patient care.

Body Techniques is structured for the convenience of the therapist, yet it retains flexibility in application since the judgment of the therapist determines the pace, intensity, and emphasis of the individual treatment session. After examining the patient, the therapist must rely on his or her judgment as to whether the treatment will concentrate on treatment of pain, corrective measures, or prevention of future episodes of pain and disability. Each phase will be thoroughly discussed in the text and illustrated with case histories. Each treatment technique with its individual components has been included because of its effectiveness in clinical application over an extended period of time. The Techniques presented have proved to be safe, easy to apply, and, most importantly, effective in assisting the therapist to achieve the goals desired for the patient.

Patients themselves are the best witnesses to the effectiveness of any treatment. For even though we, as medical practitioners, can present objective measurements and data, it is the patient who ultimately will decide whether or not he feels better and has more functional ability as a result of the treatment.

For selection of techniques to be included in *LaFreniere Body Techniques,* both of the above criteria were used. Scientifically they were determined to be physiologically sound, effective by objective measurements, and reinforced by patients' subjective reports. Reduction and eventual elimination of pain, an increase in function, and a general feeling of health, vitality, and well-being were the most common patient responses to Body Techniques.

As is protocol in other physical therapy situations, disease states as a cause of symptoms should initially be ruled out by a medical doctor so that only mechanical/functional limitations are being treated by the methods described in *LaFreniere Body Techniques.*

Joan G. LaFreniere, Ph.T.

Acknowledgments

To Ms. Annie Black, Ph.T., my associate and friend, who was the first therapist to learn and apply Body Techniques in a clinical setting.

To Ms. Gloria Stavers for choosing the title of this book, and for her professional guidance in many other endeavors.

To Ms. Barbara Robidoux for transcribing my tapes and editing the final manuscript.

To Wendelin Eve for the illustrations throughout the book.

To the staff of the Physical Therapy Treatment Center of New York for their constant striving to provide quality care and treatment of the patients entrusted to our care.

To the growing number of physicians who are exposing their patients to the benefits of physical therapy.

To the instructors at Columbia University School of Physical Therapy who instilled in me professionalism as an ideal.

To Ms. Marta Snyman for her enthusiasm for, and support of, Body Techniques.

To my many friends and patients whose support and encouragment made it possible for me to muster the fortitude to compile this material while being subjected to the constant demands of a growing practice.

Dedication

This book is dedicated to the physical therapists who continually strive to learn increasingly more effective methods of treatment to benefit their patients—and to my patients, whose devotion to Body Techniques prompted this manual.

Contents

Foreword

The manuscript is well done, and I'm sure that it will prove very useful to physical therapists and other medical practitioners applying manual therapy.

Therapeutic Touch does interface with Physical Therapy and could successfully be utilized and integrated with the Body Technique applications. For instance, to activate energy flow, instead of massaging continually, break the period of massage once circulation to the area has begun, center your consciousness and build up a field over the area and/or direct or modulate (whichever is appropriate to the situation) energies to the area for about two to three minutes. Assess area and alternate Therapeutic Touch with Body Techniques as needed for the next 5 minutes or so. This combination would seem to help speed up the results of healing.

Dolores Krieger, Ph.D., R.N.*
Associate Professor of Nursing
New York University

---

*(Author of *The Therapeutic Touch,* Prentice-Hall, Englewood Cliffs, N.J., 1979.)

Chapter 1

A Therapeutic Approach by Physical Therapy

Today's patient population is demanding that medical practitioners become more involved in a positive form of the art of medicine based on scientific fact. Patients are recognizing the fact that medicine in this century has changed from an almost entirely practical discipline to an increasingly theoretical one. This current method of medical care somehow manages to eliminate from the healing process the patient and his strivings toward the achievement of vibrant good health.

"Today's scientific medicine is in the business of bringing disease to an end. It has been in the business of death, the prevention of it, the sanitation of it, and the ritualization of it. This is a system that can neither understand nor cope with a positive notion of health, a concept wholly unto life." (*The New Physician,* March 1979, page 55.)

While we in the United States have available the most successful methods for treating acute trauma and the highest record of achievement with immunization, there is little else to prove that recipients of American medicine feel healthier, happier, or more vibrant. Nor do we know that they can occasionally achieve a feeling of well-being. As a matter of fact, the opposite is true. Even in the absence of specific disease, the general population is obese, fatigued, emotionally overwrought, depressed, anxious, unhappy, and overcome by stress-related pathologies. This situation leads us to the question that the medical community as well as the general population must face if we are to progress from a limited and often unsuccessful mode of health care: *Are we to settle merely for an absence of disease as a model of health in America?*

That we should accept so discouraging a situation is hardly probable, for even physicians are now joining patients' and other medical practitioners' efforts in search of more rewarding and health-provoking treatment techniques. The release of statistics revealing iatrogenic illnesses has forced all medical practitioners to recognize and admit the limitations of technological and pharmaceutical medicine that eliminates the human factor. One such account follows:

"... 36 percent of 815 consecutive patients on a general medical service of a university hospital has an iatrogenic illness. In 9 percent of all persons admitted, the incident was considered major in that it threatened life or produced considerable disability. In 2 percent of the 815 patients, the iatrogenic illness was believed to contribute to the death of the patient. Exposure to drugs was a particularly important factor in determining which patients had complications. Given the increasing number and complexity of diagnostic procedures and therapeutic agents, monitoring of untoward events is essential, and attention should be paid to educational efforts to reduce the risks of iatrogenic illness." (Reprinted by permission of the *New England Journal of Medicine* 304:638–42, 1981.)

Herbert Benson, M.D., Associate Professor of Medicine at Harvard Medical School and Director of the Division of Behavioral Medicine at Boston's Beth Israel Hospital, relates some relevant facts in a more personal manner. Here are some quotes from his book, *The Mind/Body Effect.**

"Unfortunately, the recent contributions of medicine have been coupled with great increases in the number of adverse complications directly attributable to drugs and diagnostic and therapeutic procedures. Whereas historically the surgeon was largely responsible for the majority of the iatrogenic complications, the medical doctor prescribing drugs has recently become the main perpetrator of iatrogenic death and disease."

"Between 3 and 5 percent of a general practitioner's patients consult him because of iatrogenic drug complications which ultimately require admission to a hospital."

"Most investigations of the iatrogenic drug problem report that between 10 and 30 percent of patients already in a hospital develop an adverse drug reaction. In one study, Dr. Leighton E. Cluff, Dr. George F. Thornton, and Dr. Larry G. Seidl of Johns Hopkins University found that 15 percent of the patients at that major medical center experienced iatrogenic effects from drugs. In another study, Dr. Elihu M. Schimmel of Yale University reported that over

The Mind/Body Effect by Herbert Benson. © 1979 by Simon & Schuster, Inc., New York. Reprinted by permission of Simon & Schuster, Inc.

10 percent of patients hospitalized experienced deleterious complications associated with the administration of drugs."

"Schimmel also found that 20 percent of patients investigated experienced deleterious complications associated with medical care. The incidence of life-threatening iatrogenic complications was approximately 5 percent of the total hospital population. The average duration of hospitalization for those who suffered iatrogenic effects was 28.7 days as compared to 11.4 days for unaffected patients."

"The current state of excessive usage of drugs and diagnostic tests and procedures is due to many interacting factors: technological advancement; commercial interests; unrealistic patient expectations; legal concerns; financial solvency of medical institutions; and reimbursement procedures for health professionals."*

In the light of these and similar statistics, responsible medical practitioners today are being forced to find alternate methods of evaluation, diagnosis, treatment, and prevention. *Body Techniques* is one such method that fits all these criteria for musculo-skeletal disorders. Furthermore, it is an appropriate mode of treatment to be delivered effectively by physical therapists.

MUSCULO-SKELETAL DISORDERS

Unfortunately, a breakdown of the previous statistics is not available to disclose how many iatrogenic illnesses took place during treatment of musculo-skeletal disorders. It is in these instances that past treatment of patients has been most shameful and unsuccessful, for drugs merely reduce symptoms and surgery rarely outperforms natural methods in restoring mechanical balance to a previously unbalanced area of the body. Physical therapists must accept their part of the blame for the past lack of success by American medicine in treating musculo-skeletal disorders because the basis of their professional training is the acquisition of the knowledge, judgment, and skills necessary to successfully treat musculo-skeletal disorders. Yet these shocking statistics continue! Consider these observations from "Musculo-skeletal Disorders: Their frequency of occurrence and their impact on the population of the United States," J. L. Kelsey, H. Pastides, G. Bisbee, Jr., *Prodist*, New York,

---

The Mind/Body Effect by Herbert Benson. © 1979 by Simon & Schuster, Inc., New York. Reprinted by permission of Simon & Schuster, Inc.

1978:

"Musculo-skeletal conditions rank first among disease groups in the frequency with which they affect the quality of life of individuals as indicated by the extent of activity limitation, disability, impairment, and handicap. About 20,000,000 people in the United States have musculo-skeletal impairments.

"Musculo-skeletal conditions rank second to diseases of the circulatory system in total economic cost, and are first among all disease groups in cost attributable to lost earnings and services from non-fatal illnesses. The total annual economic cost attributable to musculo-skeletal conditions has been estimated to be about $20,000,000,000 per year.

"Musculo-skeletal conditions rank third in frequency of occurrence among acute conditions, second in number of visits to physicians, fifth in number of visits to hospitals, and third in number of operations in hospitals."

"Musculo-skeletal conditions are not among the leading causes of death, although they are frequently involved in deaths attributable to accidents. Musculo-skeletal conditions are thus not primarily killing diseases, but are more significant in their effect on the quality of life.

"Musculo-skeletal conditions rank second to diseases of the circulatory system in the frequency with which worker disability allowances are granted and rank first in cost to workmen's compensation insurance carriers. In the United States, at least 85,000 workers receive disability allowances for musculo-skeletal conditions each year, and in California alone the total cost to insurance carriers is over $200,000,000 per year.

"Since musculo-skeletal conditions are most common in the elderly and since the number of elderly in the population is expected to increase over the next several decades, the frequency of occurrence and impact of musculo-skeletal conditions will become greater in the future, if their frequency and consequences are not reduced."

It is not enough for us to recognize the limitations in a previous system of traditional health care; we must also provide responsible alternatives. Using all of our knowledge, skill, and dedication, physical therapists must offer alternative methods of treating musculo-skeletal disorders. The need for more humane methods and what our role should be in the emergence is described in *The New American Medicine Show* by Dr. Irving Oyle (Unity Press, Santa Cruz, California, 1979):

"Caring along with . . . curing, grace . . . with gadgetry, and faith . . . produce results where technology fails." (p. 40)

"Many people are unaware . . . that they are not helpless in the face
of disease . . . they turn . . . to the health industry for help . . . to
combat what is viewed as a malevolent force which has invaded the
body . . . . Directing the patient's own defenses . . . represents an
alternative tactic." (p. 33)

We owe this effort to our patients who have often been violated by
needless drugs and surgical procedures to no avail. We owe it to the
promulgation of our profession to develop effective scientific methods of
treatment that do not exclude active participation of the patient. Finally,
we owe it to ourselves to be instrumental in change so that our existence
as physical therapists makes a difference within the health care system in
which we participate.

WHY BODY TECHNIQUES?

There is a demand today among patients and medical practitioners
alike for a method of health care which effectively incorporates physical
and psychological techniques which, in a physiologically sound way,
safely and positively affect the health and well-being of the patient. The
requirements do not stop there, however. The techniques of this health
care must be presented to the patient in a manner that 1) keeps him in an
active role throughout the therapy, 2) guides him in learning more about
his own body, 3) helps to stimulate his own healing capabilities, and 4)
will eventually allow him to be independent in his own health care except
for crisis situations. For this type of health care to be valid, three areas
must be considered: physical aspects, psychological interactions, and a
valid physiological basis.

*Body Techniques—through the Physical Aspects of Touch, Pressure,
Vibration, Stretch, and Joint Mobilization—can:*
—break up triggerpoints, nodules, and adhesions in the muscles and near
critical areas around nerves and joints which either restrict movement or
cause pain.

> "With (deep point massage) one may . . . relieve a triggerpoint . . . It
> is often combined with kneading and effleurage as a 'diagnostic'
> massage to locate triggerpoints that were hard to identify at first
> examination." (Hans Kraus, M.D., *Clinical Treatment of Back and
> Neck Pain*, McGraw-Hill, New York, 1970.)

> ". . . deep massage given to the lesion itself affords temporary
> analgesia . . . [to allow] moving the painful structure to and fro
> [whereby] it is freed from adhesions both actually present and in the
> process of formation . . . . The endeavor must be to prevent the

continued adherence of unwanted young fibrous tissue in recent
cases, or to rupture adherent scar tissue in long-standing cases . . . "
(James Cyriax and Gillean Russell, *Textbook of Orthopaedic Medicine,* Volume 2, Williams & Wilkins, Baltimore, 1965.)

—increase the range of motion of painful and/or limited joints by
mobilization and by affecting soft tissue limitations.

"Mobilization and manipulation show to best effect when directed at
mechanical problems for which they perform three main roles:
1. Restoring structures within a joint to their normal positions or
    pain-free positions so as to allow a full-range painless move-
    ment.
2. Stretching a stiff painless joint to restore range.
3. Relieving pain by using special techniques."
(Geoffrey Douglas Maitland, *Peripheral Manipulation,* Butterworth & Co. Ltd., London, Boston, Sydney, Toronto, reprinted
1980.)

—control or eliminate pain by stimulating the nervous system through
relevant mechanoreceptors.

"Though touch, pressure, and vibration are frequently classified as
separate sensations, they are all detected by the same types of
receptors. *Free nerve endings* found everywhere in the skin detect
touch and pressure. A touch receptor of special sensitivity is *Meiss-
ner's Corpuscle.* They are responsible for the ability to recognize
exactly what point of the body is touched. *Pacinian corpuscles* are
stimulated only by very rapid movement of the tissues. All the
different tactile receptors are involved in detection of *vibration,*
though different receptors detect different frequencies of vibration.
(Arthur C. Guyton, *Medical Physiology,* W.B. Saunders Co., Philadelphia, London, Toronto, 1981. p. 599.)

" . . . it will be clear that awareness of pain is not a simple function of
the intensity of peripheral nociceptive stimulation but is also related
[inversely] to the concurrent amount of non-nociceptive afferent
activity emanating from segmentally related tissue mechanoreceptors." (Barry Wyke, Neurological Mechanisms in the Experience of
Pain, *Acupuncture and Electrotherapy Res.,* 4:27, 1979.)

—increase the patient's breathing capacity for most efficient use of
bodily systems with the least expenditure of energy.

"Breathing is the way in which we transport oxygen from the air to
our body's cells, where it is used to burn carbohydrates, proteins and
fats, thus releasing the energy that keeps us going . . . breathing is

directly related in a very strategic way to the functioning of the internal organs, the emotions and the mind . . . . " (Dina Ingber, "Brain Breathing," *Science Digest,* June 1981.)

—identify areas of mechanical imbalance for future treatment emphasis.

"As we grow older, the resting state that we all learn to adopt is either a balanced or an unbalanced one, according to the degree of maldistributed muscle tension. Muscular hypertension is the residual tension and postural deformity that remain after stress activity—or after any activity that leaves behind residual muscle tension." (Wilfred Barlow, *The Alexander Technique,* Alfred A. Knopf, Inc., New York, 1973; paperback ed.: Warner Books, New York, 1980.)

—increase the efficiency of general circulation and nerve conduction by removing blocks in the body through re-establishment of mechanical balance to all affected areas.
—induce both local (to the muscle) and general relaxation effects.

". . . there is hard evidence that treatment by Therapeutic Touch . . . elicits a generalized relaxation response." (From the book, *The Therapeutic Touch* by Dolores Krieger, Ph.D., R.N. © 1979 by Prentice-Hall, Inc. Published by Prentice-Hall, Inc., Englewood Cliffs, NJ 07632.)

Is one form of Body Techniques suitable for every patient? Well, yes and no. All human beings are subject to two common conditions: stress and gravity. Body Techniques reverse the negative effects of these two sources of so much trouble so the basic treatment can benefit everyone. On the other hand, the treatment becomes individualized when it points out the areas of imbalance in each patient and helps to structure subsequent treatment protocol to eliminate the individual problems in addition to countering the effects of stress and gravity.

Stress is one of the common denominators we all share by being alive and functioning in today's world, with the complex pressures and demands it puts on the human body. Most people exhibit excess tension in skeletal muscles because of the suppression of the *fight or flight response* and because of other emotional and psychological upsets.

"Hypertension is also a result of this stress, and may give rise to many other unhealthy conditions." (Barlow, *The Alexander Technique*) "Increased activity of the sympathetic nervous system, that is, increased secretion of epinephrine (adrenaline) and norepinephrine (noradrenaline), is characteristic of the fight or flight response as well." (Benson, *The Mind/Body Effect)*

Body Techniques reverse the cumulative effects of excess stress and tension.

We also suffer the effects of living a lifetime against the forces of gravity. Some of the conditions we experience because of living with gravity are a *forward head position* resulting in malaligned cervical and lumbar vertebrae which often cause pressure on discs and nerves; tight, stiff, and unbalanced cervical and lumbar muscles because of these conditions; decreased breathing capacity because the trachea is restricted by this forward head position and the tight muscles; lack of movement in cervical, thoracic, and lumbar joints because these joints are seldom allowed to go through their normal range of motion due to malalignment; tight back muscles and weak abdominal muscles.

"That maximum extension of the skull on the atlas tends to be habitual in middle-aged and elderly people is suggested by the finding that 81% of the 300 skulls examined show evidence of osteophytosis on the posterior aspects of the occipital condyles." (R. Trevor Jones, "Vascular Changes Occurring in the Cervical Musculo-skeletal System," *S. A. Medical Journal,* May 7, 1966. p. 389.)

Gravity is a mechanical kind of stress that forces us into a posture featuring stooped thoracic area, forward head position in extension at the atlanto-occipital joint accompanied by a loss of the lumbar arch with tight low back and weak abdominal and intrinsic low back muscles. (Barlow, *The Alexander Technique.*) This posture becomes general to the population because muscular weakness increases as we become older and more sedentary. Therefore, we are not as easily able to support our bodies against gravity with correct alignment. With incorrect posture over a length of time, permanent changes become evident in joint alignment and they reinforce improper use during usual activities.

The cycle of faulty posture/restricted movement can continue to reinforce itself until conditions caused by body malalignment lead to a disease state which saps energy, vitality, and well-being. These conditions are often caused by the restricted blood circulation in affected areas of imbalance and by pathological pressure exerted on nerves to the point that their proper functioning is impeded. How can a body function properly with so many unnatural restrictions limiting its free movement, use, and enjoyment?

Body Techniques help to reverse the mechanical changes in the skeletal and muscular systems incurred by remaining upright against the force of gravity. The therapist is also able to use his or her skills in prescribing corrective and preventive therapeutic exercises to assist the patient in maintaining the corrective changes that are gained through Body Techniques.

Psychological benefits are incurred because Body Techniques:
——are delivered with the Therapeutic Touch.

> " . . . there is hard evidence that treatment by Therapeutic Touch affects the healee's [patient's] blood components and brain waves and that it elicits a generalized relaxation response." (Krieger, *The Therapeutic Touch*) Or it is delivered through the art form of Laying on of Hands (Oyle, *New American Medicine Show*) and provides all of the accompanying benefits of such an application. *The human factor is returned to medicine.*

——are delivered in a warm, caring environment with the only purpose being to increase the level of health of the patient. This atmosphere fosters the ability of the patient to develop a relationship of trust and faith in the therapist which is a necessary prerequisite for the successful application of the placebo effect.

> "The placebo effect brings us back to the human factor—the factor which ignites the healing process. Rituals like rubbing the snake-stone, laying on of hands, or prayer may also trigger the placebo effect." (Oyle, *New American Medicine Show.* See also Benson, *The Mind/Body Effect* and The Healing Brain I, course notes N.Y.C., 1981.)

——direct the intrinsic healing capabilities of the patient toward stimulation of his own immune system, thus allowing the patient to help heal himself.

> "The idea that the immune response is the body's most important defense . . . has enjoyed wide medical support over the past decade . . . unless the integrity of the immune mechanisms has been compromised. This can happen . . . under the pressure of chronic emotional stress." (*Psychology Today,* September 1980. See also Geraldine Youcha, "Psychiatrists and Folk Magic," *Science Digest,* June 1981, and Krieger, *The Therapeutic Touch.*)

——free the motor cortex of the inhibition that remains after incorrect patterns of functioning and use have persisted for a length of time.

> " . . . The faulty actions come to feel 'right' and the correct ones feel 'wrong.' The kinesthetic sense is distorted and the awareness of the body deteriorates. . . . " (Robert Masters, Ph.D., and Jean Houston, Ph.D., *Listening to the Body,* Dell, New York, 1978.)

Perhaps the most important point to be made is that Body Techniques are delivered with the Therapeutic Touch in a caring environment and that makes a whole new array of benefits available to the patient. The patient is encouraged, stimulated, and activated to learn about his own body and how to help heal it. Every person has the capabilities to heal himself. Intervention by traditional medical methods should only take place when these capabilities fail. Body Techniques will help correct existing musculo-skeletal conditions and will bring the patient's body back into balance. Corrective exercises will be prescribed to achieve this goal. Once the balance has been attained, Body Techniques along with preventive exercise and correct postural alignment can be used as a form of preventive medicine to insure life-long health.

Physiologically, Body Techniques are capable of:
—creating a transfer of human energy from therapist to patient directed toward healing with the Therapeutic Touch.

> "One such instance is the subsystem of energy which is called *prana* in Sanskrit, which my research has led me to believe to be at the base of the human energy transfer in the healing act. It does not have an adequate translation in English, primarily because our culture does not understand energy within the same context as does the Eastern world. Most often, *prana* is translated as vigor or vitality; however, an analysis of the literature indicates that the term really pertains to the organizing factors that underlie what we call the life process. *Prana,* therefore, is responsible for such phenomena as regeneration and wound healing." (Krieger, *The Therapeutic Touch.*)

—increasing the production of red blood cells which results in an increase in vitality and better general health and well-being because of the potential of raising O_2 intake.

> " . . . when ill people are treated by the laying-on of hands, a significant change occurs in the hemoglobin component of their red blood cells." (Krieger, *The Therapeutic Touch.*)

—reversing the cumulative effects of stress by continually removing excess stress tension from muscles and returning them to their resting length.

> " . . . what we have to consider is the waste of our energies over a lifetime, the effect of unnecessary tensions on our bodies over a lifetime, and the resultant damage which we do to our bodies and our lives . . . " (Masters and Houston, *Listening to the Body.*)

> "In time, not only does the resting state of the muscle become incorrectly balanced, but it begins to modify the bones and joints on which it works and also the circulatory system that traverses it. The bony framework becomes warped and cramped and stretched by the

stresses and strains that are put on it by persistent overcontraction of muscle." (Barlow, *The Alexander Technique.*)

—encouraging the release of endorphins/enkephalins through stimulation (by stretch, vibration, pressure, movement of joints, electrical stimulation (*The Journal of Orthopaedic and Sports Physical Therapy.* Volume 3, No. 4, Spring 1982, p. 204), touch, mental visualization, and the placebo effect) of dorsal root, peripheral receptors, and the hypothalamus.

"It is now well recognized that neurons containing immunoreactive beta-endorphin have a distribution in the central nervous system completely different from that of neurons containing immunoreactive enkephalins . . . In the dorsal horn of the spinal cord the central branches of primary sensory neurons enter the central nervous system. Here the various modalities such as touch, temperature, and pain are relayed to higher centers . . . . " (*Brain Peptides: A New Endocrinology,* Elsevier North-Holland Biomedical Press, 1979, eight authors.)

This release of natural opiates helps to eliminate or control pain, and hormones released are postulated to activate the immune system to encourage natural healing.

Probably the most exciting research to be published in recent years is the discovery of endorphins/enkephalins, and the postulation of how they are stimulated and released. This news is particularly relevant and encouraging to physical therapists because both the thermoreceptors and mechanoreceptors are stimulated by most of the techniques therapists use. Body Techniques is a very good example of how these treatments work clinically.

"In normal circumstances [this] receptor system is relatively (although not entirely) inactive, but its afferent activity is markedly enhanced when its constituent unmyelinated nerve fibres are depolarised by the application of mechanical forces to the containing tissue that sufficiently stress, deform or damage it (as with pressure, distraction, distension, abrasion, contusion or laceration), or by their exposure to the presence in the surrounding tissue fluid of sufficient concentrations of irritating chemical substances (such as potassium ions, lactic acid, polypeptide kinins . . . . " (Barry Wyke, "Neurological Aspects of Low Back Pain," in *The Lumbar Spine and Back Pain.*)

For some time therapists recognized the fact that touch, pressure, vibration, and stretch, along with heat and cold, worked very well in treating painful conditions, but it was not understood completely how these elements worked except for their effects on the circulatory system. Now, because of new research, we are discovering the scientific bases of how the nervous system is stimulated to work through the mechanoreceptors to release intrinsic pain-killing substances.

As reported in *Brain Peptides: A New Endocrinology: Peptide Neurons*, "Enkephalin is released at axo-axonic synapses and inhibits presynaptically the release of substance P and thus activation of postsynaptic neurons conveying impulses to higher centres . . . when these receptors are stimulated." (Costa and Greengard (eds.), "Brain Peptides: A New Endocrinology." *Advances in Biochemical Psychopharmacology*. Vol. 20, Raven Press, New York, 1979.)

This research adds a new dimension to the gate control theory of Melzack and Wall. The chemical explanation is that enkephalin is released when the dorsal root is stimulated and acts as an inhibitory agent to transmitters or modulators that carry pain signals. These data confirm the treatment modalities of physical therapists as scientifically valid and substantiate the fact that drugs rarely surpass their effectiveness for control of pain in musculo-skeletal disorders. In fact the use of drugs can even interfere with the pain-modifying chemical action of the patient's own body.

Scientific validation has finally been given to the conclusion drawn from the experiences of physical therapists. Stimulation of the thermoreceptors and mechanoreceptors by physical therapy can be effectively used to control or eliminate pain and to invoke good health and well-being. Since the methods in Body Techniques stimulate these same receptors, recent scientific discoveries also validate Body Techniques physiologically.

In addition, " . . . there is hard evidence that treatment by Therapeutic Touch affects the healee's [patient's] blood components and brain waves, and that it elicits a generalized relaxation response . . . Therapeutic Touch . . . is very good at relieving pain . . . [but] it is the patient who heals himself . . . the healer accelerates the healing process." (Krieger, *The Therapeutic Touch*.)

Therapists have always known these things; now we know why.

It can be documented, therefore, that Body Techniques aid patients in many ways. The inevitable effects of stress and gravity can be relieved. Physical problems resulting from malalignment or bad habits can be corrected. The patient can become the agent of his own healing and gain the confidence necessary to reach new levels of good health and well-being. Both patient and therapist can take advantage of the body's natural pain-fighting substances to eliminate or control pain without the use of drugs. First and last, Body Techniques only heal; they induce no iatrogenic disease.

"Unfortunately, the recent contributions of medicine have been coupled with great increases in the number of adverse complications directly attributable to drugs and diagnostic and therapeutic procedures." (Benson, *the Mind/Body Effect.)*

Body Techniques presents a safe and effective method of treatment that will be of great benefit to many patients.

Chapter 2

Body Techniques System

The five areas of treatment form the core of Body Techniques, consisting of seven parts which include thirty-eight different movements. Together with modalities and therapeutic exercises they provide a thorough evaluative review and a flexible system through which a wide variety of patients' problems can be treated. For the convenience of the therapist, a worksheet of these Techniques appears on page 51.

Body Techniques can be useful as a diagnostic method as well as a mode of treatment. An important procedure which should be constantly utilized by both patient and therapist is the comparison of a structure on one side of the patient's body to the same area on the opposite side. Is a muscle on one side stiffer or more tender than on the other side? Is the mobility, flexibility, texture, thickness, or bulk of the muscle group different from its counterpart? Is movement of a joint painful and/or lacking in range of motion on one side but not on the other? These comparisons should be made throughout the application of the Body Techniques system.

It is important in all Body Techniques to fit the style of treatment to the physique of the patient. While it may require all the strength the therapist can muster to treat a heavy, muscular person, it is equally possible that a judicious, light touch will be needed for more fragile patients. The therapeutic touch and practice will guide the therapist, but it is important to remember to take the side of least harm in case of doubt.

The following contraindications should be observed by the therapist when considering the applicability of the therapy.

Local Contraindications for Performing Body Techniques

- Recent or unhealed fracture
- Dislocated/subluxed joint
- Extreme muscle spasm of unidentifiable etiology
- Open skin lesions
- Radiating pain exacerbated by any Body Technique

General Contraindications for Performing Body Techniques

- Extreme dizziness
- Nausea (severe)
- Blurred vision
- Tinnitus (in combination with other signs)
- Flu, virus, severe cold (initial stages)
- In the presence of any acute systemic disease

Indications for Performing Modified Body Techniques

- Mild signs of vertebral artery compression (with proper precautions)
- End stages of flu, virus, common cold
- Acute radiculopathy (any level)
- Acute muscle spasm
- Deconditioned state
- Moderate/severe psychological disturbance

BODY TECHNIQUES—PART I

The patient begins the treatment lying prone with hands at sides, comfortably supported by pillows. (One under the patient's abdomen to support the lumbar curve; one under the anterior aspect of the lower legs for comfort). The therapist should be positioned, possibly on a low stool, with sufficient height to allow both hands to rest comfortably on the patient without either overly bending the elbows or stretching the arms. Therapists practicing these Techniques will find that they need to employ their own body weight and leverage as well as arm and hand power if they are to treat more than one or two patients a day.

Soft powder is used instead of lotion so that the therapist's hands can feel the underlying structures without the gliding-over motion caused by the use of lotion. Sprinkle powder along the spine and smooth it over the back with a light circular motion. At the beginning of the treatment, the therapist uses a stroking movement which starts at the base of the patient's neck, continues down one side of the vertebrae, then back up the other. This gentle movement accustoms the therapist and patient to each other, allows the patient to relax, establishes rapport and atmosphere, and prepares the patient for the more serious movements. At this time, the therapist begins to direct all attention and energy to the patient; the patient uses this time to become accustomed to the therapeutic touch of the therapist. His thinking should follow the hands of the therapist and their breathing should be in unison whenever possible.

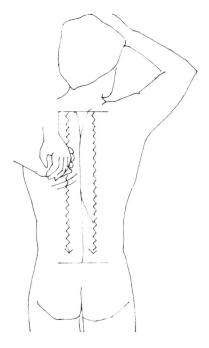

Figure I-a

I-a. *Fingers on transverse process; pressure with vibration*

Starting at the bottom of the neck or at the beginning of the thoracic vertebrae, the fingertips of the therapist's dominant hand are placed on the transverse processes of the thoracic vertebra and gentle downward pressure is exerted with a vibratory force; this pressure is assisted by the therapist's other hand, which goes on top of the knuckle region of the main hand. Both hands exert a downward and vibrating pressure on the transverse processes of the thoracic vertebrae all the way down to L5 on one side of the spine; then the hands slide back to the upper thoracic level of the other side of the spine to repeat the process.

The purpose of this Technique is to loosen both the superficial and the deep layers of muscles, to palpate for existing triggerpoints or nodules, and to test for muscle spasm or tightness and muscle imbalances as noted in comparison with the other side of the patient's body.

Technique I-a also affects the costovertebral joint, which connects the vertebra and the rib. Gentle vibratory pressure: 1) encourages increased movement of this joint; 2) informs the therapist as to whether or not the rib cage on that side is rotated by its position and by the amount of spring in the rib cage. When the fingertips are on the costovertebral joint, the palm of the hand is more toward the lateral aspect of the rib cage; and as the therapist presses down and vibrates with the fingertips, the fingers and palm can feel how much bounce there is in the rib cage and whether or not it is rotated. 3) identifies rotated vertebrae easily.

I-b. *Therapist's hands on posterior aspect of ribs, crossed and spread apart*
Pressure is downward and outward in a lateral motion away from the spine. The patient should exhale in unison with the pressure exerted.

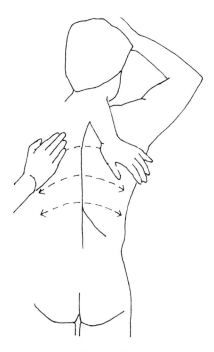

Figure I-b

This Technique also allows the therapist to test the rotation of the rib cage and to encourage a more natural placement of the rib cage at the costovertebral joint.

I-c. *The therapist's forearms are on the sacrum and the lower thoracic area*
Stretch in opposite directions to extend muscles and joints that are usually stiff and tight in the lower back area.

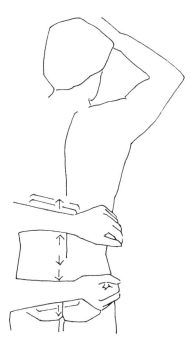

Figure I-c

This Technique produces gentle, natural movement in an area of great restriction in many patients. It also prepares the lumbar vertebral area for more advanced Techniques to come later, namely acupressure with the patient in a sitting position.

The therapist is informed by this Technique of the degree of stiffness in the lumbar area in general and if the lumbar area tends to move as a unit or individually by the amount of stretch that takes place. If there is very little movement available, the therapist should continue to evaluate by performing the "pinch and roll" technique to determine whether or not fibrositis is present.

BODY TECHNIQUES—PART II

The patient moves to the supine position with one pillow under his knees for comfort, none under his head. The therapist has both feet on the floor for maximum traction and stability.

II-a. *Arm-pull from behind head of table*
  The therapist draws the patient's arms, held firmly at the wrist, to one corner of the table. The amount of tension in the patient's neck

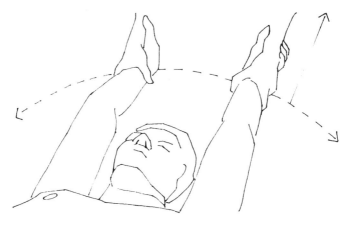

Figure II-a

and the general tension he is experiencing can be determined by
whether or not the patient's head rolls to the side the therapist
moves to. If the therapist moves the patient's arms to the right
corner and puts a traction pull on them and the patient's head stays
facing directly up to the ceiling, there is an indication of excess
tension in the head and neck area, and the therapist knows that the
patient is not completely relaxed. In this case, encourage deep
breathing until the patient's head drops to the side of the stretch. If
the same movements are made and the patient's head falls to the
right, the therapist knows that the patient is more relaxed and is
responding favorably to the initial phase of Body Techniques.

When the therapist supports the extended arms over the patient's
head and there is an increased distance between the treatment table
and the patient's shoulder on one side, it is clear that the shoulder
has decreased range of motion. The therapist should evaluate
further and use this information to set up a corresponding exercise
program to increase the range of motion of the shoulder or shoulders
or include mobilization in subsequent treatments if the joint is
limiting motion. Relief of shoulder protraction is also necessary if
the patient's head is to return to the natural, relaxed-head position.
This is a necessary prerequisite for normal body alignment.

This maneuver (II-a) encourages general relaxation, stretches the pectoral and deltoid muscles, and relieves the tension in the shoulder area in
general. It is not a specific Technique but rather a general Technique
used to induce and measure relaxation and for judging the amount of
tension in the patient's neck and body. It also helps to relieve muscle
tension and tightness from the upper back, the scapula, the shoulders,

and the arms and neck in general. Notice also during this Technique if the patient is lacking in range of motion of anterior flexion of the shoulders. This is often the situation with people who have protracted shoulders from exaggerated head position over a long period of time.

II-b. *Shoulder depression with vibration from behind head of table*
Standing behind the patient's head, the therapist gently pushes the patient's right shoulder down using one hand cupped over the top of the shoulder. A slight vibration is added at the end of the stretch to help relax the muscles. Then the left shoulder is pushed down and vibration applied. By alternating sides, the therapist can determine how much tension and restriction there is at the neck and shoulder region. If the right shoulder is depressed and the patient's head rolls to the right, the therapist will know that there is abnormal tightness and restriction at the right occiput and/or right cervical musculature. It is important for the therapist to note whether the patient experiences pain during this Technique and whether it is on one side or both. Also, by noting whether the shoulders can be depressed the same amount or whether one side moves more freely than the other, the therapist gains information to add to the assessment of whether any imbalance exists.

This Technique checks the general flexibility of the area and the resilience of the structures involved: the trapezius muscles, the anterior and posterior cervical muscles, movement of the clavicle, and the shoulder girdle in general. It also promotes general loosening of an area

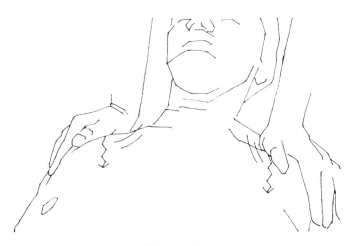

Figure II-b

where most people accumulate excess tension from stress and postural strain.

The shoulder depression is a good example of the purposes and uses of Body Techniques. All of these Techniques help the patient regain natural movement. Some are specific for certain muscles or joints, but most are general in that they help the therapist identify areas that need additional treatment. The shoulder depression Technique assists the therapist in uncovering additional information about the neck and the shoulder girdle so that future treatments can concentrate on the areas that need correction. Through observation, touch, comparison, and patient symptomatic explanations, the therapist and patient work together to improve the patient's condition.

II-c-1. *Head wobble*

Standing behind the patient, the therapist places her hands on each side of the patient's head and wobbles it from right to left with the back of the patient's head remaining on the table throughout.

This exercise encourages general relaxation and rotational movement from side to side. Its object is to test the cervical range of motion generally and to help assess the flexibility of the musculature. It also teaches the patient how to roll his head effortlessly, letting gravity take the head from side to side without undue effort. This Technique is carried through in later exercise programs to assist in correcting the forward head position by encouraging the use of the head and neck

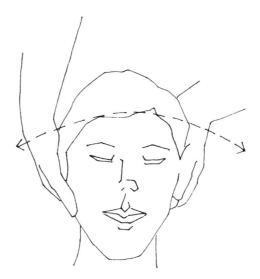

Figure II-c-1

independently of shoulder muscles and for increased proprioceptive awareness of the position of the head and neck. It also prepares the patient for the next two Techniques, as it encourages general relaxation and loosens the muscles on the anterior and posterior aspects of the neck.

To add the shoulder push to this Technique (see II-c-2), the therapist places the left hand on the patient's right occiput and the right hand on the patient's right shoulder. The opposing stretching movements here will help stretch the sternocleidomastoideus, which exhibits excess muscle tension and lack of normal flexibility in about 90% of patients. Elimination of restriction in the sternocleidomastoideus and other cervical musculature at the neck allows the patient the necessary range of motion to attain proper head position by the end of the treatments. Thus a series of Body Technique treatments helps the patient attain proper postural alignment by releasing restrictions which allow for the relearning of proper proprioceptive positioning of the head.

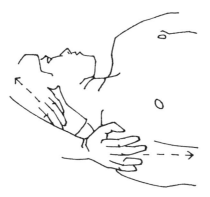

Figure II-c-2

A further maneuver in this Technique is occiput pressure with stretch (II-c-3 and II-c-4). After the muscles are substantially loosened from the head wobble and added shoulder push, the therapist takes the patient's head in both hands, index and middle finger of each hand at each side at the occiput. The patient's head is laterally flexed to one side (II-c-3). As the neck is stretched toward the left side, the patient's head is turned so that the pressure of the head rests on the therapist's right index and middle fingers (II-c-4). The fingers vibrate the head slightly so that there is pressure and vibration on the right occiput using the weight of the head to add to the pressure. This movement encourages normal range of motion at the atlanto-occipital joint by stretching the heavy band of ligaments that attach the cervical vertebra to the occiput. It is worth

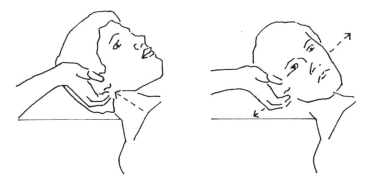

Figure II-c-3   **Figure II-c-4**

noting that 90% of the patients who seek therapy for neck and back pain exhibit restriction or abnormal tightness at this joint. (Clinical statistics, New York Physical Therapy Center, 1160 Park Avenue, New York, New York 10028.) The therapist is looking for gentle shifting of soft tissue just inferior to the occiput bone when this Technique is done; in many cases there is no movement initially. Either the joint is locked and/or the muscle attachments/ligaments around the joint are so tight that normal motion is prevented. This Technique will, with time and repeated treatment, loosen the soft tissue and allow proper range of motion of the joint. The Technique itself evaluates the general mobility of the area and checks the condition of the soft tissue that surrounds it. This Technique, and others aimed at the atlanto-occipital area, encourages forward flexion at the joint where the majority of the population become fixed in varying degrees of extension as a normal aging consequence. It is important to note that sometimes a restriction is unilateral at this point. If so, we would most likely expect to find other limitations on the same side of the body throughout Body Techniques. (Remember that the patient is to be held in slight flexion throughout the cervical Body Techniques. Avoid allowing the head to fall back into extension at any time.)

II-d. *Lateral flexion*

Standing behind the patient, the therapist holds the back of the patient's head slightly off the table and in slight flexion with the right hand. The left hand goes as far down the patient's neck as possible. Using a gliding motion with both hands, the therapist moves the patient's head and neck all the way to the right until lateral flexion is felt at the inferior cervical vertebra. With the therapist's superior hand, the patient's head is laterally flexed to the left side while the inferior hand remains fixed at that level. The movements are repeated until the atlas is reached.

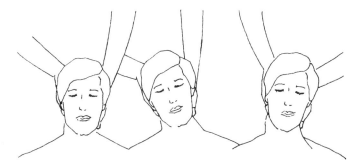

Figure II-d

This Technique reveals if there is any limitation in lateral flexion at any level. Sometimes application of the Technique alone will bring the joint into proper alignment since lateral flexion is the primary action of these joints. As a matter of fact, this happens quite often in practice especially since the prior Techniques have loosened the cervical muscles.

It is important to ask the patient if there is pain in a restricted area at a given level, as *the patient's symptomatic reports are always important* in evaluation. If there is restriction, the therapist will put the emphasis of the remaining Body Techniques on those that affect the cervical area. If the pain or restriction is persistent, a more specific mobilization Technique may be used.

II-e-1. *Vertebra pressure with rotation*

The therapist holds the patient's head in a slight flexion with the right hand. The left hand is placed as far as possible down the neck, to C7 or C6, depending on the patient's anatomy. When the left hand is at the lowest level possible with the particular patient, the head will be rotated from side to side. When rotating the patient's face to the right, the therapist's right index finger will be putting a lifting

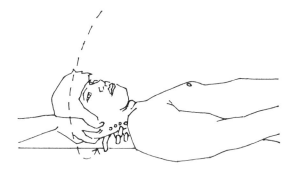

Figure II-e-1

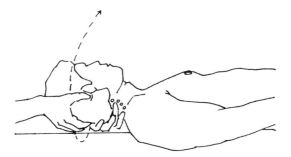

Figure II-e-2

pressure on the right side of the vertebra. Remaining at the same level, rotate the patient's head to the left (II-e-2). The therapist's left thumb will be putting pressure on the left side of the same vertebra at the transverse process. The therapist moves the left hand slowly up the cervical spine, gently checking the rotation of each vertebra. If there is a limitation, sometimes this movement alone will free it. If not, the Technique may be repeated several times or another specific Technique may be used in combination.

II-f. *The Nod*
The therapist holds the patient's head in slight flexion with her right hand at the occiput and the left hand on the forehead. As both inhale/exhale, the therapist exerts a traction pull with the right hand and a downward force with the left hand. Together these multi-directional forces result in a "nodding" action at the atlanto-occipital (OA) joint which encourages its increased range of motion.

II-g. *Cervical stretch*
The therapist puts one hand under the patient's occiput and the other one on the patient's forehead. The knuckles of the bottom hand stay on the table. The patient's head is put in slight flexion. Both therapist and patient inhale and exhale together during this

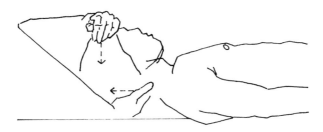

Figure II-f

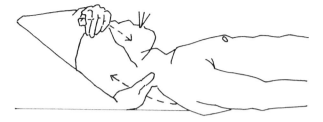

Figure II-g

Technique to coordinate their strength and energy. The therapist uses body weight to put traction on the patient's cervical area.

BODY TECHNIQUES—PART III

The patient sits in a firm, straight-back chair, arms at sides, facing the treatment table.

III-a. *Scaleni and superior angle of scapula vibration with breathing*
     The therapist puts one index finger just above the clavicle, where the scaleni and sternocleidomastoid attach. The thumb of the same

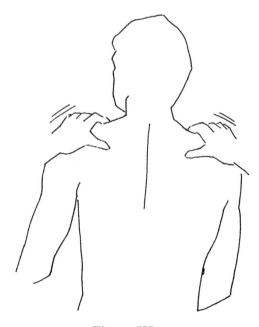

Figure III-a

hand reaches over the shoulder and rests just medial to the superior angle of the scapula. Pressure with vibration is put on both areas simultaneously while the therapist rests the palm on the shoulder. First one side is pressed, then the other, then both together to compare. The patient will be the first to tell you whether he feels a numbing, tightness, tenderness, or discomfort on one side more than the other. Repeat two or three times on each side, until the muscles begin to loosen.

If there is tightness on one side, it usually indicates that: 1) the patient's muscles are overworking to hold the head in the forward head position; or 2) that you will find from other Body Techniques that there is also a corresponding limitation on the same side at the atlanto-occipital joint, shoulder area, or with scapular movement.

III-b. *Deltoid massage along teres*
    The therapist places a thumb at C7 on both sides and begins to pick up the trapezius muscle. The therapist continues all the way along the shoulder using thumb pressure on the supraspinatus along the way to the distal aspect of the deltoid muscle. At the muscle, from the shoulder joint to its insertion, pressure is applied and released with a "pinching" action. The deltoid muscle is not stretched during normal daily activities so there is often a buildup of tension there

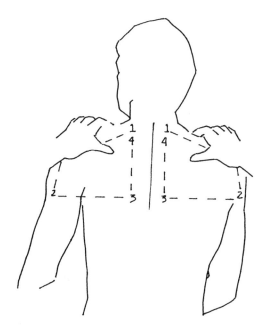

Figure III-b

especially when the shoulder musculature is used to support the head and neck. Squeezing the deltoid is also very relaxing generally to the patient. After the squeeze, the therapist can run the fingers into the teres major and minor muscles and return to C7 in a sort of circular movement. Two or three circuits will be necessary to cover the area sufficiently.

III-c. *Clavicle lift*

The therapist's hands rest on the patient's shoulders, the forefingers hooked under the clavicle starting at the sternum. The thumbs rest on the patient's back and act as stabilizers while the therapist uses the fingers to put a lifting, rolling pressure on the underside of the clavicle to give an upward motion. This Technique releases the tension in the pectoralis muscles. It also encourages natural movement in the joints at either end of the clavicle, where it attaches to the sternum at one end and continues to form the acromioclavicular joint at the other.

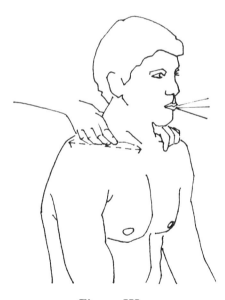

Figure III-c

III-d. *Occiput to shoulder massage*

The patient sits in a firm straight-back chair placed near the edge of a table high enough so that he may rest his head on his crossed hands comfortably on one or two pillows. Standing behind the patient, the therapist, using the thumb and forefinger of each hand at the same

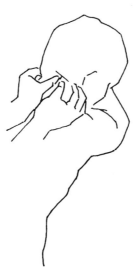

Figure III-d

time, applies a pinching-type motion deep under the occiput so that the tendons and ligaments that attach at the occiput are picked up and moved.

The atlas is most often restricted in cases of neck pain when these structures limit range of motion of both skeletal and soft tissue movement. The muscles are not able to move through their full range of motion because of this joint restriction, so it is not surprising that they become very tight and painful. When the condition has existed over a long period, the patient will feel pain when this Technique is first applied because the area has not moved normally for some time.

It is best to start with a light pinching motion, trying to get as far underneath the occiput as possible, and then working inferiorly along the posterior cervical muscles from the upper trapezius to the shoulder. This Technique is repeated two or three times. Its purpose is to release all the tension in the muscles treated, to loosen the structures that are limited in motion, and to induce a deeper level of relaxation as all deep cervical techniques do. The therapist also compares one side with the other to see which one is tighter and more painful to the patient so that further treatment can be concentrated where it is most needed.

III-e. *Occiput with shoulder pull*

The patient's head is positioned with forehead down on forearms on pillows so that the neck is arched as much as possible. The therapist places the left thumb on the patient's right lateral occiput. At the

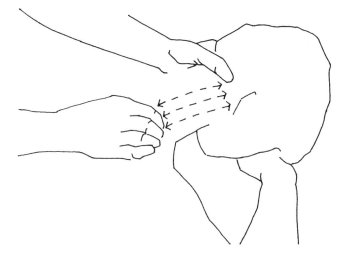

Figure III-e

same time the therapist lifts the posterior aspect of the muscle with the right hand and with an opposing motion of pushing the occiput away and lifting and pulling the corresponding muscle, he or she performs a deep stretch. The left thumb is moved inward about a half an inch on the occiput and the right hand is moved correspondingly to pick up the next most medial part of the muscle. This movement is repeated until the midline is reached. The therapist then returns to the areas in which the muscles were difficult to pick up and the Technique is repeated. The same movements are repeated on the other side with the therapist's right thumb on the patient's left occiput, the left hand picking up the sets of cervical muscles on the outside of the neck. The pressure of the thumb and fingers going in opposite directions stretches the muscles and begins to loosen restricted joints.

This Technique begins to give more range of motion to affected soft tissue and joints in the area, especially the atlanto-occipital joint that is often very tight and restricted. Again, the emphasis is on restoring normal range of motion and balance of one side against the other. Getting the sides to have the same flexibility, the same range of motion, and the same pain-free movement in both the muscles and joints will eventually lead to normal and pain-free function.

III-f. *Occiput drilling*

The therapist's open hand travels up the patient's neck until the open fingers arrive at the occiput. The outstretched fingers will be

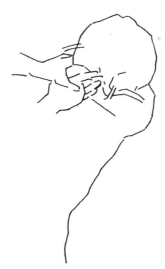

Figure III-f

underneath the occiput as the therapist vibrates the hands and pushes forward in a direction that encourages forward flexion.

Because of the position of the patient's head (slight flexion), this Technique helps to loosen the atlanto-occipital joint and the ligaments that attach on the occiput by producing a motion that they usually do not have a chance to perform when the patient is locked on this point backwards into extension.

III-g. *The Nod, sitting*

The therapist places both thumbs directly on each side of the occiput. She leans her body weight forward into her thumbs to produce the "nodding" motion at the OA joint and continues to apply pressure for approximately 6 seconds. This Technique is repeated two to three times, to reinforce the increased range of motion gained through previous Body Techniques.

Caution: The thumb pressure should be relieved between individual "nods" to avoid vertebral artery compression.

III-h. *Thumb vibration along spinous processes*

With the patient in the same position as for III-g, the therapist places one thumb on either side of the vertebrae beginning at C7 and, exerting pressure with the side of one thumb and then the other, works back and forth deeply down the back (alternating on both sides of each spinous process) to the sacrum.

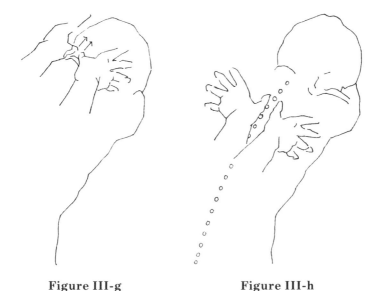

Figure III-g   **Figure III-h**

This friction movement loosens the deep muscles and tendons along the vertebrae. Also because there is vibration and pressure it helps to loosen restricted vertebrae and gently align them to encourage natural range of motion of the joints. As the therapist works along the vertebrae, it will be clear which ones offer more resistance, which muscles are tighter, if there are any myofascial nodules or triggerpoints, or if there are immobile areas of vertebral-segments that don't respond equally. The therapist will then be informed about areas which need extra emphasis, either by specific techniques for mobilization or particular attention during Body Techniques.

BODY TECHNIQUES—PART IV

The patient is sitting in a chair with head on crossed hands on pillows.

IV-a. *Acupressure above the iliac crest*

The therapist moves both hands down to the area above the iliac crest. One thumb is placed just above the iliac crest, midway between the spine and the outside of the body on either side. Both the therapist and the patient inhale and the therapist leans forward so that body weight aids in putting pressure on the area for 1 to 3 seconds, alternating sides, until the underlying structures begin to "let go."

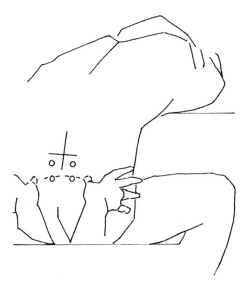

Figure IV-a

This pressure helps to release the excess tension and encourages stretch in the paraspinal muscles, tendons, and ligamentous structures that attach on the iliac crest. Again, it is important to compare one side with the other. Is there more muscle bulk on one side? If so, the side with increased bulk would indicate either the presence of muscle spasm or an increase in muscle strength. Further investigation is necessary. Is there pain on one side but not the other? If so, future treatment will concentrate on the painful side. The therapist will make a mental note of the reactions of the two sides and of how this information supports other pertinent data about the patient's condition collected from prior Body Techniques.

IV-b. *Acupressure along transverse processes of spinal vertebrae to C7*
The therapist moves the fingers into the lumbar vertebrae just above the sacrum. One finger rests on each transverse process of the same vertebra (for the lumbar area) and reverse pressure is applied on *one side at a time.* For instance, if pressure is applied by the left thumb on one side of the spine, when this is released, reciprocal pressure is applied by the right thumb on the other side of the spine in a rocking-type movement. Each application of pressure should last from 1 to 3 seconds. The procedure is repeated two to four times, depending on the amount of resistance felt. If there is a great deal of resistance or tightness, a more specific evaluation and treatment by advanced mobilization/manipulation Techniques can be performed

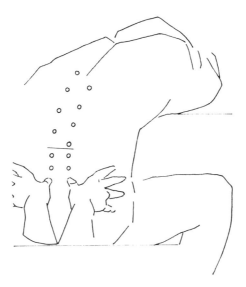

Figure IV-b

by the therapist. If the patient complains of pain or tenderness, and if the therapist feels that the muscle consistency is thicker or bulkier, more vibration is added to the pressure and the procedure is given a few more times to release the resistance.

This procedure is repeated until the bottom of the rib cage is reached. At the thoracic area, the levels of the thumbs change—on one side of the body they will be at one level and on the other side they will be at a level about a half-inch above the other hand. This change in thumb placement is necessary to encourage rotation because the shape and direction of movement of the thoracic vertebrae change. As the hands move up to the thoracic area, their main job is to assist in rotation of the vertebrae. Pressure is applied on one side and then on the other in the same rocking manner that will encourage this rotation. During the process, the thumbs will be on different levels. As one thumb is moved up, it is going to approximately be a half-inch above the other one on the other side of the spine. Continue this action all the way up the spine to C7 (the large bulge at the base of the neck) and at that point apply slight friction with the thumbs around the spinous process of C7.

This is an important Technique and should be done carefully. The therapist needs to use total concentration for correct placement of the fingers on the transverse processes. Concentrate on what is felt and seen, always checking one side of the body against the other. Try to feel the consistency of the muscles and joint movement while watching the patient's reaction. Listen to the patient's comments and complaints. If there are segments of the spinal column that seem to be immobile, note the areas for future treatment. It is also important to note the distance between the vertebrae (spinous processes). Marked differences may indicate that two or more vertebrae are not moving freely of each other. The purpose of this Technique is to release soft tissue restriction along the spine (including the deep muscles and tendons that attach there) and to encourage joint range of motion. If there is limitation of movement, often this Technique is enough (in conjunction with other Body Techniques) to loosen the restrictions. If the therapist finds that after several treatments there is still limitation of movement between two or more vertebrae, he or she may want to do more specific mobilization/ manipulation techniques at a level identified through the Phase structure of the Body Techniques program (see Chapter 3).

During Techniques IV-c, d, e, and f, the patient sits upright on a firm straight-back chair with arms at sides.

IV-c. *Acupressure at superior angle of scapula*

The therapist's thumbs are placed just medial to the superior angle of the scapula. This is a point at which many elements attach: tendons and multiple layers of muscles. It is a good release point for these structures. Both the therapist and the patient inhale and exhale while the patient leans back on the therapist's thumbs. As they both exhale, the therapist applies pressure and vibration. The patient should lean back onto the therapist's thumbs with as much force as is comfortable while exhaling, about six seconds in most cases.

The purpose of this Technique is to release all of the tension in this area and also to encourage scapula movement. As always, the therapist should compare the sides of the area, checking for restrictions, if both sides are at the same level, and if both sides offer similar resistance. This maneuver is done only once.

IV-d. *Acupressure along medial border of scapula*

The patient is still upright, arms at sides. The therapist applies pressure with her thumbs downward along the medial aspects of the scapula bilaterally at the same time to produce the "rocking" motion. If there is great resistance and/or tightness in the structures the therapist can apply pressure while the patient pushes backward into her thumbs.

This pressure also releases the tension in the muscles that attach on the scapula. This is an area that often has an accumulation of triggerpoints,

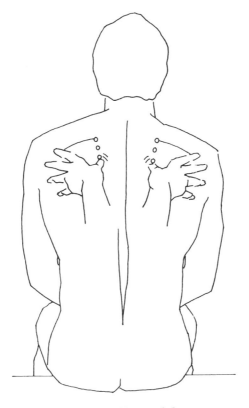

Figure IV-c and d

especially if there is a limitation of cervical, shoulder, or scapular movement. Excess tension, spasm, or triggerpoints may form, also, if a patient has experienced an injury or chronic pain at any of these joints.

IV-e. *Acupressure with elbow on trapezius with cervical rotation*
   The therapist's position is at the side of the patient and at 90 degrees to him. The therapist's left elbow is on the trapezius muscle where the greatest bulk is, a bit closer to the neck than midway. The thumb of the right hand is at the left occiput. Both patient and therapist inhale, and as they exhale, the therapist lets his or her weight bear down gently with vibration on the trapezius, with an occiput push and a slight rotation of the head. The movement of the head is on a diagonal rather than a straight plane, a corner to corner action.

This rotating movement releases excess tension in the sternocleidomastoideus and upper trapezius, loosens ligamentous structures that attach

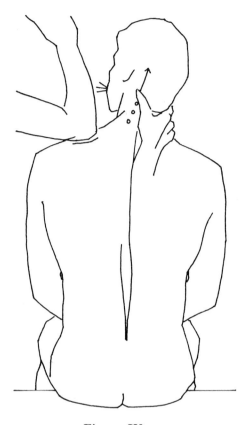

Figure IV-e

at the occiput, and encourages natural range of motion of the neck at the atlanto-occipital joint. The elbow pressure at the trapezius releases the tension in the shoulder muscles. It also depresses the shoulder girdle which aids in relaxing and readjusting the deep structures of the shoulder. Repeat on opposite side.

IV-f. *Acupressure lift on the occiput*

> The therapist puts a thumb on one side of the patient's occiput, a forefinger on the other, with his or her elbow on her iliac crest of the pelvis for support. The therapist's other hand goes on the patient's forehead and both patient and therapist inhale and exhale as the therapist lifts the patient's occiput straight up into cervical flexion, which encourages traction at the atlanto-occipital joint.

This is another way to encourage motion at the atlanto-occipital joint, apply deep relaxation to the muscles and tendons that attach at the

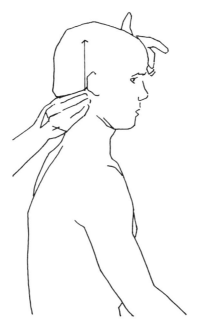

Figure IV-f

occiput, and the muscles of the neck. This Technique is very relaxing to the patient because it is a movement that helps to relieve the tension accumulated during normal daily activities and especially from holding the forward head position because of faulty posture. The patient should actively tuck his chin during the "lift."

BODY TECHNIQUES—PART V: POSTURAL ADJUSTMENTS

The patient sits erect in a firm straight-back chair, arms at sides.

V-a. *Shoulder depression with forearm; added cervical rotation and stretch*
Standing at the patient's side, the therapist rests a forearm on the trapezius muscle of the patient midway on the shoulder (not at the end of the shoulder since it is not the purpose of this Technique to apply acromioclavicular pressure). The thumb of the other hand goes at the occiput and the forefinger around at the other side so that the therapist is holding the back of the patient's neck in the hand. Both therapist and patient inhale and exhale while the therapist puts gentle pressure down on the trapezius muscle rather

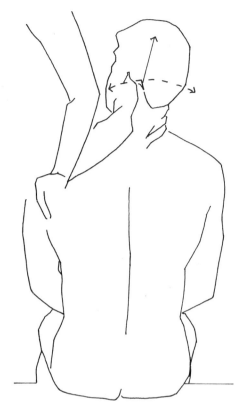

Figure V-a

than on the forward plane of the clavicle. The thumb puts pressure upward on the occiput and slightly rotates the head so there is a stretch on the sternoclavicular and other anterior muscles, especially those strained by the forward head position. Some of the posterior muscles as well are affected. The therapist adds a slight vibration at the end of this pressure.

This Technique reverses the effects of bad posture due to gravity. Because of the forward head position posture, many patients have a great deal of tension in the trapezius muscle and the sternocleidomastoideus and anterior muscles which pull bony segments into extension. This Technique encourages a stretch and natural range of motion in the cervical joints and muscles and a downward depression of the shoulder girdle. It helps to loosen restricted muscles that are forced to hold a faulty posture of the head and neck.

V-b. *Rib cage rotation to one side*

One of the therapist's hands is on either side of the patient. The left hand holds the left shoulder of the patient so that it doesn't move; the right hand will be on the back of the rib cage pushing forward against the holding pressure of the left hand. This motion resembles opening a door.

The rotation encourages range of motion at the thoracic vertebrae and encourages the correct positioning of the rib cage. Patient and therapist should exhale with the push.

V-c. *Scapula pull*

The therapist stands on the side at a 90 degree angle to the patient. The patient puts his arm in the small of his back so that the rhomboid muscle relaxes. The therapist puts his or her left hand on the front of the patient's shoulder; the fingers of the right hand are placed under the inferior angle of the scapula. The therapist and patient inhale and exhale together. As they exhale, the therapist lifts the right hand to try to stretch the muscles that attach on the inferior angle of the scapula. Then the right hand moves up slightly while the left hand vibrates the shoulder so that the fingers can get underneath the scapula more easily. The therapist uses body weight

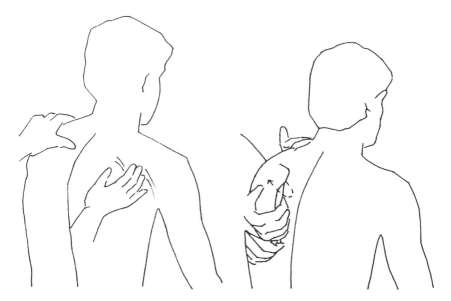

Figure V-b   **Figure V-c**

and leans backward to pull the scapula with vibration away from the patient's body.

This is a standard mobilization technique for the scapula, but instead of its being done with the patient prone, it is applied sitting up for convenience and general application. The purpose of the Technique is to encourage normal range of motion of the scapula and to attain the proper flexibility of the muscles that attach on its medial aspect. These muscles often are affected by chronic forward head position, postural strain of shoulders, long periods of scapula stabilization, and strain because of muscle weakness. Most patients who demonstrate a cervical or shoulder dysfunction have a problem at the scapula where it joins the thorax. This Technique helps to correct the problem. Should the limitation at the scapula remain after several treatments, mobilization in the side-lying position can be added to the therapy.

V-d. *Scapula push with patient rotation to the opposite side*
The therapist stands behind the patient and slightly to the left. The therapist's left hand is on the front of the patient's left shoulder. The therapist's right hand is on the scapula with the fingers pointing toward the ceiling. The therapist exerts a push-pull pressure: the right hand pushes and the left pulls the patient's body toward the therapist. Both therapist and patient inhale and exhale together. The patient rotates toward the right from the waist simultaneously with the therapist's action.

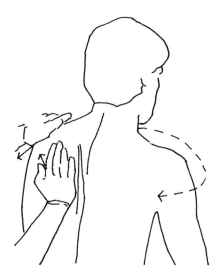

Figure V-d

This Technique encourages natural range of motion at the costovertebral and sternocostal joints, while aligning the general position of the rib cage.

BODY TECHNIQUES—PART VI: SPRAY AND STRETCH

The patient sits upright in a firm straight-back chair, hands at sides. The spray and stretch technique is well documented in the literature of physical therapy. It incorporates spraying a vapor coolant over the skin covering a muscle that is tight or in spasm, thereby enlisting the neurological reflex arc in helping the muscle to relax. In other words, the spray is used once, twice, or three times along the length of the irritated muscle, using only enough spray to act as a counterirritant. The spray cools the skin above the muscle, the neurological system picks up the stimulus and, through a reflex arc, the appropriate motor nerve is stimulated to relax the tense muscle.

VI-a-1. *Head drop to one side with spray*

The patient's head should drop comfortably to one side. The therapist's hand cups the ear on the side to which the head drops (VI-a-1). Tell the patient there will be a cool spray, then slightly turn his or her head and with the other hand spray ethyl chloride on the lengthened muscle beginning at the occiput and continuing along its body to the distal attachment. It usually takes two or three sprays to adequately cover this area. Remember to spray in one direction only and instruct the patient *not* to inhale deeply while, or directly after, spraying.

After spraying, the therapist's right forearm is placed across the patient's right shoulder. By cupping the patient's left ear with the right hand the therapist gets a firm hold on the patient's head (VI-a-2). A slight pressure is put on the trapezius and shoulder with

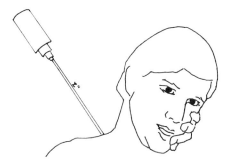

Figure VI-a-1

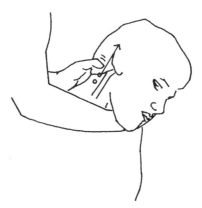

Figure VI-a-2

the right forearm. With the left hand, the therapist applies pressure with the thumb at the right occiput. By slightly rotating the wrist, there is even greater stretch to the sternocleidomastoideus and the trapezius and the other musculature of the neck. Next, the therapist asks the patient to inhale and exhale slowly while the therapist maintains a firm hold on the head. The patient should be entirely relaxed with the therapist holding his head up. The command is, "Make your head as heavy as possible while exhaling." Stretch and rotate the head slightly with a gentle vibratory pressure added.

This Technique is very relaxing. If there is a great deal of tightness in the patient's neck or if the patient's original problem area was the neck, the therapist could continue with the third part of this Technique.

The right hand slightly lifts the patient's head. With the left thumb, move down the different vertebrae in the neck and add a slight rotary pressure by moving the right and left wrists concurrently. After the original lengthening is done and the ethyl chloride is sprayed, the therapist will slightly raise the patient's head with the right hand and then will take the thumb and move downward on successive vertebrae gently applying pressure with the thumb while adding a rotary movement with the wrist. This movement can be done to approximately C5 depending on the patient's anatomy. Repeat each Technique on the other side and compare reactions.

VI-b. *Bend-Sit with spray or ice; roll down and up in segments; add pressure and stretch*

The patient turns around in the chair so that his back is in front of the therapist and the back of the chair is to his left. He should sit upright and with good posture while inhaling deeply. He slowly

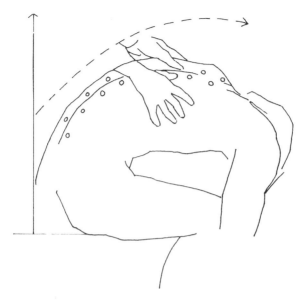

Figure VI-b

begins to exhale, tucks the chin in, and with hands between knees, slowly rolls down vertebra by vertebra. The therapist puts two fingers on either side of each vertebra and in doing so helps the patient gain body awareness to achieve a slow rolling down so that he can roll over as far as possible without stress to the lumbar area. If the patient has difficulty rolling down, he should be told to roll down like a rag doll by becoming very limp and loose and relaxing vertebra by vertebra. When the patient is completely rolled down, the therapist tells the patient that there is to be a cool spray. The therapist starts to spray at C7 and continues down the right side of the spinal column and then repeats on the other side. While the patient is still rolled over, the therapist puts her fingers on either side of the spine at L5-S1 and applies pressure to the paravertebral muscles and slowly progresses up the spine with the side of the thumbs (VI-b).

This Technique helps to add stretch to the paravertebral muscles and encourages firing of the mechanoreceptors as explained in Chapter 1.

The therapist returns to the lumbar area with open hands and puts some pressure on one side of the back and then the other, all the way up the spine (VI-b-1). The weight of the therapist is used to relax the muscles that are further away from the spine and also to help encourage forward flexion at each vertebral level.

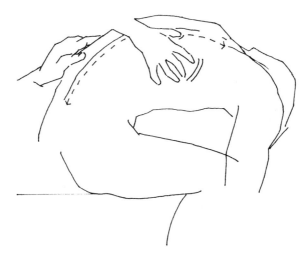

Figure VI-b-1

This maneuver helps gain more movement of the vertebral joints of the spinal column and relaxation of the attached muscles.

Now the patient should roll up slowly (VI-b-2). Instruct the patient to pull up as much as possible with his stomach muscles while exhaling. When he is about one-third of the way up, instruct him to

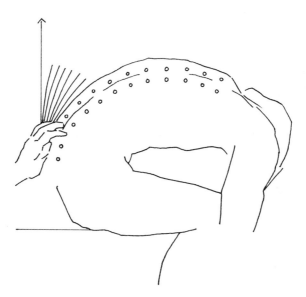

Figure VI-b-2

let the lower back muscles take over, then later the upper back muscles. The shoulder musculature should be relaxed throughout. When the patient is fully upright, the therapist can apply slight pressure to the mid-thoracic area to help the patient adjust his head to the proper position. The therapist completes this Technique by adjusting the patient's head by putting a slight pressure under the occiput with the right hand while holding the forehead with the left. The head should be brought back and upward. One Bend-Sit has now been completed. Another is usually done without the spray. If the patient's back is exceptionally tight or if he is recovering from a muscle spasm, the spray would be used a second time.

BODY TECHNIQUES—PART VII

The patient sits on the side of a firm chair with his back to the therapist.

VII-a. *Pectoralis stretch with breathing and vibration*
The therapist places one knee at the edge of the chair and the patient is instructed to round his back against the supporting knee. The small of the patient's back should press against the therapist's knee as this allows for greater stretch at the shoulders. The patient puts both hands behind his neck and clasps the fingers. The therapist takes the patient's elbows in his or her hands and asks the patient to inhale and to exhale slowly as the therapist gently opens and lifts the

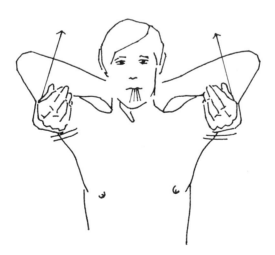

Figure VII-a

elbows. Special care should be taken so that the patient does *not* push his neck or head into a forward head position during this Technique. The process is repeated twice more while carefully monitoring the patient's reactions. *Note:* In the sitting Techniques in which the therapist is behind the patient, it is helpful, in gauging the patient's reactions, to have a mirror placed so that the therapist can see the patient's face.

This Technique provides a productive stretch on the patient's chest and shoulder musculature. Slight vibration at the end of this stretch further enhances its effectiveness. The Technique helps reverse the protracted shoulders and relieves the tensions that develop in the chest and shoulder muscles from leaning over a desk, walking with a forward head position, or from merely standing upright against the pull of gravity. Extreme caution should be used if the patient has a chronic dislocating shoulder.

VII-b. *Head alignment with awareness of spine alignment*

This Technique, which patient and therapist do together, is designed to allow the patient to experience increased proprioception of correct head placement. It should make the patient more aware of how important it is to use the abdominal muscles to support the head in its proper position on the neck and shoulders.

The patient sits on the side of the chair, back to therapist. The therapist puts her thumb and index finger on either side of the occiput; the forearm of the therapist must be along the patient's

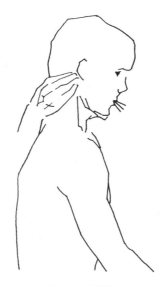

Figure VII-b

spine. The patient is instructed to inhale and to exhale slowly as he pushes the *back* of his neck only into the therapist's fingers. Most patients will bring the head back by bending at the neck, or push the head back by throwing it into extension at the neck. To counteract this, the patient is instructed to tuck the chin in and then to push the neck back again. After three or four repetitions (while the therapist puts pressure on the back of the head and aids correct position with the forearm on the spine), correct head position is achieved unless the patient has extremely tight cervical musculature. In that case, the Technique will be reserved until further treatments have loosened the involved muscles. Sometimes the patient will begin to push back on the therapist's forearm with the upper spine. He should be instructed, "Don't push with your back, only with the back of your head." The therapist should continue to instruct the patient: "Now tuck your chin in; push your head back; tuck your chin; push your head back. Feel what is happening to your spine." At the end of the exercise, ask the patient if he feels his stomach pull in. Ask, "Do you feel your spine align?" "Do you feel anything happening in your lower back?" "Is your stomach pulling in?"

The object of these questions is twofold: 1) to give the patient the experience of knowing what it feels like to have the head in the correct position (sometimes after the patient is put in the correct head position, the therapist extends him at the atlanto-occipital joint to show him that the weight distribution changes as the position of the head changes in space), and 2) to bring to the patient's attention that correct head position and spine alignment result from the stomach being pulled in, not from tight shoulders. The patient may be asked to relax his shoulders and wiggle them so that he can see that correct head position is not dependent on rigid shoulders, very likely one of the reasons that got him in trouble in the first place. The correct head position is held by reversing the thoracic stoop and by pulling in the stomach muscles (and having strong stomach muscles to pull in). The patient should be exhaling during the entire push, as this Technique becomes an isometric exercise. Usually this Technique needs to be done only once, until the patient achieves correct head position. If he does not on the first try, it should be repeated. You may also give corrective exercises along with Body Techniques to help the patient achieve correct head position on his own (see Chapters 3 and 4).

The entire series of Body Techniques requires approximately 20 minutes to apply effectively for a general session. If an area of concentration is included, an additional 5 to 10 minutes is required. Since Body Techniques was never meant to be the entire therapy exclusive of other methods, it is always preceded by a modality to enhance the therapy's effectiveness and completed by the addition of corrective exercises prescribed by the therapist. If the correction has already been accomplished and the patient feels no pain or lack of function between treatments, then Body Techniques may be combined with preventive therapy, usually including a combination of flexibility and strengthening exercises. This regimen is described in detail in Chapter 3.

BODY TECHNIQUES SYSTEM WORKSHEET

Part I—Prone
  a. Gentle vibratory pressure on transverse processes of thoracic vertebrae
  b. Pressure on posterior aspect of ribs
  c. Sacrum and lower thoracic area stretch
Part II—Supine
  a. Arm pull from behind head of table
  b. Shoulder depression with vibration from behind head of table
  c-1. Head wobble
  c-2. Head wobble with shoulder push
  c-3,4. Occiput pressure with stretch
  d. Lateral flexion
  e-1,2. Vertebra pressure with rotation
  f. The Nod
  g. Cervical stretch
Part III—Sitting
  a. Scaleni and superior angle of scapula vibration with breathing
  b. Deltoid massage
  c. Clavicle lift
  d. Occiput to shoulder massage
  e. Occiput to shoulder pull
  f. Occiput drilling
  g. The Nod, sitting
  h. Thumb vibration along spinous processes
Part IV—Sitting in a Chair with Pillow
  a. Acupressure above the iliac crest
  b. Acupressure along transverse processes of spinal vertebrae to C7
  c. Acupressure at superior angle of scapula
  d. Acupressure along medial border of scapula
  e. Acupressure with elbow on trapezius with cervical rotation
  f. Acupressure lift on the occiput
Part V—Postural Adjustments
  a. Shoulder depression with forearm; added cervical rotation and stretch
  b. Rib cage rotation to one side
  c. Scapula pull
  d. Scapula push with patient rotation to the opposite side
Part VI—Spray and Stretch
  a-1,2. Head drop to one side with spray
  b. Bend-Sit with spray or ice
  b-1. Pressure and stretch Bend-Sit
  b-2. Roll down and up in segments
Part VII—Sitting on side of firm chair
  a. Pectoralis stretch with breathing and vibration
  b. Head alignment with awareness of spine alignment

Chapter 3

Theory of Application

Body Techniques is a manual therapy program which is both evaluative and corrective. It is used as the base for each patient's treatment program because it is a vital force in the treatment of pain, provides touch information for continuing patient evaluation which outlines protocol for subsequent treatments, and is a major factor in the correction of underlying dysfunction. Body Techniques is the system of manual technique illustrated in Chapter 2 and the complete therapeutic approach to patient treatment as capsulized in the chart on page 78. Although this program is standardized in presentation, in application it is as highly individualized as is each patient's musculo-skeletal profile. Therefore, entry into the program is made at a stage which is specific and personalized. The accurate evaluation by the therapist of the patient's presenting areas of concern and the continual reevaluation of patient progress is vital to the application and success of the total program.

INITIAL EVALUATION

Communication

The Initial Evaluation provides an opportunity for the therapist and patient to establish the relationship of trust and cooperation that is essential for a successful outcome to the therapy. In considering the patient who confronts the physical therapist daily, we find it likely that his pain has proved intractable to medicinal or surgical intervention and is chronic in nature so that he is not only hurting but is also discouraged. Physical therapy may truly be his last chance for relief. Since success can be achieved only through trust and cooperation between patient and therapist, it cannot be stated too strongly that this initial communication during the evaluation is extremely important, as it sets the tone of all future interaction. Encouraging the patient to express his symptoms and concerns, i.e., when he feels pain, which functional activities he is limited in, and what has helped alleviate or exacerbate the discomfort, aids the therapist in forming an impression of the situation that purely clinical examination might not. Remember that at this stage the patient knows more about his body than the therapist can possibly know; therefore, we must learn from him. Communication at this introductory level establishes the trust necessary to expedite the transmission of vital information from therapist to patient when it becomes crucial in the later stages of treatment.

Rapport Building

For physical therapy to be successful, it is imperative that the patient have full faith and trust in the therapist. The trust and rapport necessary must be developed at the Initial Evaluation and reinforced at each visit or whenever possible during the program. Maintaining an unhurried, caring, and sympathetic atmosphere at all times is essential for this type of nurturing. Soliciting and responding to patient accounts of pain and its easing will produce benefits to both because the therapist will learn about the condition of the patient from the one who knows best how the treatment is progressing and the patient will participate and remain active in his own treatment by coming to know his body and how it functions. As the treatments progress, the therapist prepares the way for the patient to assume increasing responsibility for his own treatment by educating him about his condition and his body.

Evaluative Information

What information should be derived from the Initial Evaluation? A Patient Profile should be compiled which includes:

1. The formal medical history and diagnosis, if any.
2. The patient's subjective description of pain and an interpretation of his functional limitations, i.e., pain during functional activities; movements that lessen or increase pain; comfortable and uncomfortable rest and sleeping positions; reaction to recreational activities.
3. The patient's subjective report *during* the Body Techniques application at the Initial Evaluation in order to assist the therapist in discovering any mechanical imbalances that may be present, including when pain occurs during specific and gross movement.
4. The results of the physical therapist's Therapeutic Touch evaluation.

Levels of Treatment Priority

To ascertain the levels of priority for treatment, the therapist should:

1. Check for *mechanical imbalances* using all traditional measurements (ROM, MMT, etc.) in areas of concentration.
2. Make a *functional assessment* by checking the integration in movement and function of all areas; ascertaining what symptoms are exacerbated by which movements; and discovering which positions or movements cause or relieve pain. The information gained reveals which structures are involved and in what plane of movement.
3. Evaluate patient's *postural alignment* with mobility tests as well as in static positions, because postural malalignment may be the first clue to serious structural and functional abnormalities. For example, having the patient bend from the waist, from side to side, with arms held over the head will allow the therapist to compare lateral trunk muscles bilaterally. Extreme pulling pain or tightness on one side will usually indicate weakness on the opposite side and restricted motion of low back and hip on the same side. Such results would indicate two areas of concentration, both of which would require further specificity testing.
4. Ascertain the *duration* of the condition. This information is important in forming the treatment approach. For instance, for a more chronic problem, the Treatment of Pain Phase would be shorter and the Corrective Phase of therapy would be longer and sometimes rather painful in itself. Knowing what is likely to be required by way of treatment helps the therapist to explain the protocol to the patient so that both will develop *realistic expectations.*
5. *Listen to* and *watch* the patient. Initially, listen without interruption to whatever he has to say, for as long as it takes him to describe adequately what he is feeling, then ask necessary questions. Watch the patient for facial expressions or unequal or sluggish performance while he is moving, bending, changing positions, etc. His reactions will give clues to the structures involved because the manner in which a patient sits, stands, and changes positions often reveals postural compensations he is making for otherwise unobserved, underlying dysfunctions. Encourage the patient to be active in describing his pain by asking him to let you know of any pain he may feel during any part of the evaluation examination, i.e., when the pain appears, when it disappears, intensifies, etc. The same instructions should be given throughout the entire program of treatment since the information it gives the therapist is important.

During the Corrective Phase, the pain is literally being "chased" by the treatment and its location and intensity help to identify underlying areas for future concentration by exposing which deeper structures and/or movements are involved.

In an Initial Evaluation of this nature, the therapist uncovers the information necessary to enable the correct placement of the patient in the multifaceted and ongoing Body Techniques treatment program (see page 58). At the same time, the patient is apprised of his condition and the role he will play in his own treatment. In summary, then, the Initial Evaluation should:

1. *Identify* the etiology of pain or the area(s) of pain.
2. *Expose* the area(s) of primary concentration for treatment.
3. *Place* the patient in the scheme of treatment for the therapist.
4. *Develop* realistic expectations for the results of the treatment program in general.
5. *Outline* the physical therapy program for both the patient and the therapist.
6. *Define* areas of responsibility for the patient and the therapist and begin the interaction between the two which is necessary for healing.

Patient Education

It is important to the success of the treatment that before the patient leaves the Initial Evaluation he knows generally what his problem is. The explanation of it should include three levels: the *neuromuscular* system, the *skeletal* system, and the *functional* implications as related to the patient's problem. He should be cognizant of the nature of his problem and its effect on the interrelation of these three areas; of how his particular problem developed mechanically; and of what the possibilities are if the condition remains untreated. If the patient has any additional health problems as described by his doctor, medical history, etc., these also should be included in the discussion.

The educative aspect of the Initial Evaluation will be much more effective if the therapist will suggest a test or movement that allows the patient to feel the limitation in the painful area. For example, if the patient has a right low-back problem, it is useful for him to do a movement that lets him feel pain, tightness, pulling or restriction on that side. But when he repeats the movement on the left side he will not feel the same sensation of pain, pulling, tightness, or lack of movement. The therapist can use this demonstration or explain why there is pain on one side but not the other and how this relates to the overall dysfunction.

What muscles are involved, which skeletal structures are affected, and the functional results of these situations can be easily explained in a manner the patient can relate to. This three-level approach (neuromuscular, skeletal, functional) has proved most effective in helping patients understand the need for treatment and explaining their responsibilities in its success.

At the conclusion of the initial session, the therapist should make a clear statement of what the therapy will encompass. Now that the Initial Evaluation has given the therapist the information necessary to establish the patient's point of entry into the treatment scheme, the total program can be explained with the aid of a schematic such as the following:

Treatment of Pain	Correction	Prevention

This type of diagram aids the therapist in formulating and structuring the therapeutic treatment. It also presents a pattern of treatment progression by which patient and therapist alike can easily understand the protocol. In addition to explaining *what* the patient may expect, it is important to give him an estimate of *how long* each phase of treatment may take. The therapist should stress that time estimates are based on experience of similar cases but that they are by no means certain. Providing reliable additional information of this kind goes a long way in establishing rapport between patient and therapist. Individual treatment methods should also be discussed elucidating the reasons for choosing one method over another. Discussion of *why* the therapist is using heat or ice, Ultrasound, or low-volt electricity will help the patient understand and cooperate with his own treatment. He should be schooled in advance as to what manual work is involved on the part of the therapist and the effort and time required for the home follow-up portion of the therapy. Of course, the patient should be encouraged to ask questions at all stages of the Initial Evaluation.

Any printed material the therapist can provide will also be helpful to the patient but should *never* replace personal interaction. If a therapist finds that the patients being treated are falling into categories of ailments, it might be helpful to prepare some printed guidelines (with plenty of room for written changes) to supply to each, as they may be able to absorb the written material better at home than from the discussions in the office in what, at best, must be a time of considerable stress.

TREATMENT OF PAIN PHASE

Most patients will enter the Body Techniques program in this initial phase. Patients who have recent pain of any duration or pain which can be easily duplicated but may not be actively experienced at the moment of a visit enter treatment at the beginning of the treatment pattern, i.e., the Treatment of Pain. The therapist should explain that generally this phase of treatment consists of ice applications, electrical stimulation, pulsed Ultrasound combined with electricity when needed, manual work, Body Movements, and very gentle exercises. The patient should also be informed that he will be instructed to follow through at home with the ice treatments and the prescribed exercises. Ice will be applied every time pain is felt and twice a day, whether or not pain is felt, to be followed by the gentle Body Movements prescribed. It is imperative that the patient realize that his participation at home is crucial to the successful outcome of the therapy, and that if he does not follow instructions, the results of the treatment will be mediocre at best.

In the beginning phase of treatment, ice and Body Movements are used as alternatives to drug therapy. While the treatment of pain is a basic and vital element of Body Techniques, not all patients enter treatment with pain. Those who do not are people whose problem is of a more chronic nature or those who are experiencing residual mechanical problems from a previous acute attack or traumatic incident. These patients, therefore, would enter treatment in the Corrective Phase. Also entering treatment in the Corrective Phase are patients (about 15% of all patients) who experience pain only periodically, i.e. once a month, twice a year, etc., yet who are bothered enough by functional or mechanical problems to seek treatment.

Classifying which patients will begin in which phase of treatment is an essential preliminary responsibility of the therapist because the goal and plan of each sector of the treatment is different. Therefore, for proper planning of techniques and realistic goal setting, this initial categorization is necessary. The proper phase of entry is determined by the dysfunction and the symptoms a patient is experiencing at the time of the Initial Evaluation. A further breakdown of the treatment scheme shows the importance of correctly classifying patients' dysfunctions and/or symptoms.

Treatment of pain		Corrective		Preventive
acute	subacute	chronic	restorative	maintenance

ACUTE STAGE

Most patients who have pain, even if it is in only a small part of the area of concentration, will begin treatment in this stage of therapy. The most common conditions to be treated are pain of unknown etiology but related to movement, muscle spasm, triggerpoints, and inflammation and neurological irritation of soft tissue structures.

Example

If on Initial Evaluation a patient has severe cervical muscle spasm (underlying fractures, disease, etc., eliminated by x-ray or other diagnostic tests), exaggerated by faulty posture and muscle weakness, and intensified by emotional stress, he would fall directly into the acute stage of the Treatment of Pain Phase. Strengthening the weak muscles initially would be contraindicated, as it would intensify the spasm. In so doing it would make it virtually impossible to interest the patient in holding himself in a healthier posture since he would be suffering intense pain. The object of his initial treatments, therefore, would be to decrease the pain and muscle spasm and reduce emotional tensions so that the patient could progress to the Corrective Phase for treatment of the underlying condition. These goals are accomplished through a combination of cryotherapy, low-volt electricity, light applications of Body Techniques (especially those performed with the patient prone with vibration and gentle rotation of the head), and careful and sympathetic attention by the therapist to the patient's response.

The *goals* of the acute stage of the Treatment of Pain Phase will be:

1. To decrease or eliminate pain.
2. To release the spasm and tight muscles enough to examine underlying tissues and structures through the application of Body Techniques.
3. To bring the patient to a point of decreased pain so that he will develop trust and faith in the therapist and in the program of treatment. This goal especially instills motivation to continue through the other phases of treatment and engenders hope for a full recovery.

If the patient is advised during the Initial Evaluation that the goal of the first two to three weeks of treatment will be to eliminate or substantially decrease the pain and this goal is met in the projected time, the patient will develop a trust in the credibility of the therapist and will form positive attitudes and expectations. Therefore, the information and time estimates given by the therapist during the early days of treatment are especially important.

The *treatment components* most often used in the acute stage include:

1. Modalities
   a. Low-volt electricity
   b. Cryotherapy (ice massage and ice packs)
2. Body Techniques (especially those that include breathing, relaxation, acupressure, and vibration)

3. Body Movements
4. Home Instruction
5. Education/Information

It is very important that the patient have full confidence and faith in the therapist from the onset of treatment. Therefore, the therapist must strive to continually make the patient feel confident, positive, and secure in his therapy. One step in the accomplishment of this goal is the instruction in proper home application of cryotherapy. Ice should be applied whenever prescribed movements or exercises produce pain or whenever pain is felt whether during exercising sessions or not. This education in pain management allows the patient to control his condition independently, improves the situation in general, and gives him the tools to utilize should his neck or back "act up" or "go out" again.

The following guidelines for *home application of ice* should be given to the patient at the conclusion of treatment session one.

Your Home Treatment*

"Adequate treatment of an acute muscle spasm requires attention several times a day. Therefore, in order to augment the physical therapy treatment you receive, we are supplying you with the following instructions for the Ice Massage and exercise."

Why Is Ice Used In Your Therapy Program?

"When a muscle is in a shortened state and painful, it influences nerves in the area and the muscle can go into spasm (a painful contraction). Ice is used so we can return the muscle to its natural resting state without causing more pain, which will lead to more spasm, etc. It is a vicious cycle that we can break with ice."

Ice Massage

"Fill 4 oz. paper cup three-quarters full and put in freezer until frozen. When ready to use, tear off about one inch of the cup so that some of the ice is showing while the bottom of the cup can be used to hold onto. Massage the entire muscle area as instructed by your therapist. You may use circular or up and down strokes, but do *not* hold the ice in one spot."

*This and the following four sections are reprinted from *The Low-Back Patient* by Joan G. LaFreniere, Masson, New York, 1979, pp. 75–76.

There Are Four Phases To The Ice Massage:

"1. Cold   which you feel when you first apply the ice
"2. Ache   after a few minutes
"3. Burning   After about 5 minutes it will feel like your skin is
               burning. At this point, remove the ice for a minute
               or so.
"4. Numbness   THIS IS THE CRUCIAL PHASE. Return the
               ice and massage until all the burning disappears.
               This signals the end of the ice massage.

"Now the ice massage is completed. The entire procedure should take 5 to 7 minutes. Do *not* massage more than 7 minutes for a small area or more than 10 minutes for a large area.

"An alternative to this method is to use a plastic bag filled with ice cubes. Wrap ice-filled plastic bag in a thin wet towel and place it over area indicated by the therapist. Keep in place for 20–30 minutes following criteria listed above under four phases to ice massage."

Exercise

"Now you can very gently move the tender muscle by following the exercises prescribed by your therapist. Do not perform any sudden, jerky movement, or do more exercises than the number and repetitions given to you. Should you feel any pain while exercising, use the ice for another minute or two, until the pain disappears. You should feel no pain while exercising.

"Repeat this procedure three times (3×) a day."

The ice is left on the painful area as long as possible to control pain and to make it easier to exercise the affected muscle without further exacerbation of pain. It is impossible to indicate exactly how many minutes the ice should be left in place because of the great number of variables that come into play. Each patient differs in skin texture, amount of fat under the skin, and muscle bulk. The therapist and the patient must cooperate during cryotherapy to effect numbness over the entire affected area. The ice is removed when the patient informs the therapist that numbness is felt. If there is still pain, the ice can be returned for a minute or two until a burning sensation is felt at which point it must be removed immediately to prevent damage to the skin.

These instructions apply to patients who have normal sensation. Therapist should be cautious with patients who have had prior surgery because their sensation may not be intact. Extra care should also be taken with older patients or with areas of patients' bodies where circulation may be compromised. The general contraindications for cryotherapy should be followed.

Muscle Spasm

Relieving muscle spasm is very important in treating musculo-skeletal conditions as it is often a cause, or result, of pain.

"It is known that pain stimuli can cause reflex spasm of local muscles, which presumably is the cause of much, if not most, of the muscle spasm observed at localized regions of the human body. Any local irritating factor or metabolic abnormality of a muscle—such as severe cold, lack of blood flow to a muscle, or overexercise of the muscle—can elicit pain or other types of sensory impulses that are transmitted from the muscle to the spinal cord, thus causing reflex muscle contraction. The contraction in turn stimulates the same sensory receptors still more, which causes the spinal cord to increase the intensity of contraction still further." (Arthur C. Guyton, *Medical Physiology,* W.B. Saunders Co., Philadelphia, London, Toronto, 1981. p. 638.)

This is most successfully accomplished with applications of Body Techniques, ice, and electrical stimulation. Whether a patient has muscle spasm as an acute problem exclusively or as an acute symptom of a chronic condition, he begins treatment in the acute stage of the Treatment of Pain Phase. The main goal is to break the muscle spasm in order to relieve the pain without exacerbating the underlying condition if there is one.

If the patient is suffering from muscle spasm that is moderate to severe, the painful area should be frozen first. If the spasm is mild, *electricity* can be used first.

"Groups of muscles in spasm due to minor injury or secondary to strain, chronic postural fatigue, or arthritic conditions may be stimulated for the purpose of relaxation. This, in turn, gives relief of pain and freedom of motion." (William J. Shriber, M.A., M.D., *A Manual of Electrotherapy,* 4th ed., Lea & Febiger, Philadelphia, 1975.)

Example

If the pain is on the right side of the low back, two electrodes would be put directly over the painful area as long as both electrodes are on the same muscle. Two electrodes would also be placed over the identical group of muscles on the opposite side, in this case the left low back. It is often the case that when one side is in spasm and is painful the other side is stiff also. If the painful side is released, the other side being unaccustomed to the new movement on the affected side, may as a result go into spasm. The current applied to break a muscle spasm will begin with five to fifteen minutes of low tetanizing current which will fatigue the muscle.

A muscle in a steady state of contraction (spasm) can be relaxed, without aggravating the condition, by fatiguing it. Ice applied to a serious spasm slows down the velocity of the stimuli returning to the spinal cord long enough for the tetanizing current to fatigue the muscle without causing it to revert to the spasm state. After fatiguing the muscle with tetanizing current, 15 minutes of a low surging current can be given in order to limber the muscle and help it respond correctly and more naturally to the kind of stimuli it is most likely to receive in normal functioning. After the muscle is relaxed, gentle Body Movements along with Body Techniques can be applied to assist the affected muscle in maintaining its resting length. (See "Effects of Ice on Nerve Conduction Velocity," J.M. Lee, M.P. Warren, S.M. Mason, *Physiotherapy,* January 1978, Vol. 64, No. 1.)

The *Body Techniques* that work best in the treatment of muscle spasm are those that apply pressure to and around the area of spasm and those that add a vibratory motion after pressure has been applied. These Techniques help to release the muscle spasm by working through the patient's own nervous system. A very slight lengthening (a return to its resting length) of the muscle that is still cold or frozen can be tried as this is an effective way to break the spasm. If the spasm is severe and is not relieved by these Techniques, the therapist can very carefully add a spray and stretch technique with ethyl chloride or ice massage with the muscle in a stretched position (taking extra care not to cause a burning sensation of the tissue since its resistance has been lowered by previous ice applications).

In the treatment of muscle spasm, the patient *must* follow through at home to reinforce the efforts of the therapist. Regardless of the severity of the spasm, the patient is instructed to go home after treatment, apply ice packs to the area, and then execute the gentle Body Movements prescribed. Because the muscle has been tight and shortened for an extended period, it will immediately revert to the shortened and painful spasm state if the patient calls upon it to work normally or if he makes any quick movements with it. Therefore, instruction should be given that home pain control consists of ice application to the same degree of numbness experienced during the office treatment.

Body Techniques

When a patient is suffering from mild, moderate, or severe muscle spasm, the general goal of Body Techniques during the acute stage would be to apply some pressure and vibration to the affected muscle and surrounding musculature. There should be no heavy stretching as that would have a tendency to neurologically induce the muscle to return to its short and painful position. Therefore, a *modified* application of Body Techniques would be indicated, as it would successfully assist the tightened muscle that is in spasm to return to its resting state through appropriate stimulation of the mechanoreceptors (see Chapter 1).

Since Body Techniques need not always be applied *in toto* (and indeed sometimes should not be), it can be broken up into its component parts for modified application. *Components of Body Techniques for clinical application throughout all phases of treatment are:*

1. Light application of all or some Techniques
2. Moderate application of all or some Techniques
3. Heavy application of all or some Techniques
4. Application with patient prone
5. Application with patient supine
6. Application with patient sitting
7. Spray and stretch techniques
8. Breathing/relaxation
9. Information/education
10. Attitudinal formation
11. Feedback from the therapist to provide motivation and encouragement

Auxiliary components to be used in conjunction with Body Techniques include:

1. Specific joint mobilization/manipulation
2. Soft tissue mobilization
3. Therapeutic movements, exercises
4. Conditioning exercises
5. Postural alignment during treatment and functional activity
6. Modalities: high- or low-volt electricity, pulsed Ultrasound with electricity, heat, cold, and laser biostimulation

Body Movements versus Therapeutic Exercises

It is important early in the therapy to distinguish between the Body Movements presented in detail in Chapter IV and therapeutic exercises so that the patient will understand the importance of performing such simple "exercises." Body Movements gently move a body area whose movement is restricted either because of an underlying chronic condition or as a symptom of it. They encourage range of motion of joints and will eventually allow limited muscles to return to their natural resting state. Body Movements also provide the initial proprioceptive awareness for patients who must relearn the correct position of the head, pelvis, and spine for proper posture. They *do not* strengthen or stretch muscles, correct any underlying condition around the joint or in the muscles, or correct any mechanical imbalance.

A therapeutic exercise, on the other hand, either stretches a limited muscle, strengthens a weak muscle, or significantly changes the area in some way mechanically. *Causing major mechanical changes in the area is definitely contraindicated when a patient is in pain or while his muscles are resisting change by remaining in spasm.* In this case, it is desirable to begin to induce natural movement and range of motion with Body Movements. This is postulated to stimulate the nervous system to release endorphins (see Chapter 1) which helps physiologically in controlling the patient's pain in a natural manner.

When the patient understands the difference between Body Movements and exercises, he must then learn what movements he will have to do at home following his treatments. It is vital that the patient know in advance of his obligation to follow through at home (once or twice a day and whenever pain is felt) with ice therapy and gentle Body Movements to reinforce the benefits received from the therapist's treatment. This home therapy will keep the patient active in his health care, allow him an increased level of control over his pain, and progress him more quickly through the treatment scheme.

Additional Information Retrieval

Once normal motion is established, the therapist must guard against a tendency to overlook the patient's subjective reports. The necessity of listening to patient complaints remains valid throughout all phases of the therapeutic program. If the patient reports pain only in one position or that it increases or decreases or does not appear at all under certain circumstances, the therapist must use this information as a clue in the detection of underlying dysfunction. At times, the patient's subjective reports will be the only means of discovering the presence of an underlying dysfunction. Most often though, these reports will substantiate the conclusions that the therapist has arrived at from checking the patient thoroughly, applying Body Techniques, and specific testing to discover new areas of concentration for treatment. Ideally, all three retrieval methods (patient report, checking through Body Techniques, results of specific tests) will be used.

To gain information vital to successful therapy, patient feedback is crucial throughout all phases of Body Techniques. Therefore, one of the primary duties of the therapist is to constantly encourage good communication and to strive for open interaction. Listening to what patients say and continually testing and pointing out changes during the performance of Body Techniques and additional tests are ways to accomplish this purpose. With this approach, the patient is allowed to assist the therapist in correctly interpreting clinical assessments. Does the motion feel the same to him on each side? Does pressure on the right and left side feel the same? Is one set of muscles tighter or more restrictive than the other? These questions should be asked constantly and the therapist must incorporate the patient's responses in future decision-making regarding treatment direction.

How much a patient can help the therapist depends greatly on how in touch he is with his body and how much body awareness the patient has developed through his life experiences. Patients who have a high level of this awareness make the therapist's job much easier because they are able to report the necessary information, i.e., what they are feeling and what changes are taking place. For patients who have not used their bodies extensively and do not have a high level of awareness, the therapist must continually point out the physical changes taking place and do more of the work of evaluation and analysis. When working with the less-aware patient, there is a need to question constantly, listen, and interpret correctly what the patient communicates, even though it may seem not to apply to the treatment or is not the direct reply to a question that the therapist is expecting.

It is important to accumulate all possible information before formulating the treatment plan for any particular session. Decisions on whether to use ice or heat, the placement of electrodes, the type of electricity to be given, and the emphasis of Body Techniques are all based on what the patient relates concerning his condition since the last treatment and what the therapist gathers through the various information retrieval methods. *The therapy program is constantly adjusted and readjusted by what the therapist sees, feels, and measures combined with what the patient can contribute about his own condition.*

Adjustments in the Program

When pain remains the same after several treatments, some variables which may lead to a change in the treatment protocol must be considered.

If the therapist was diligent in gathering and interpreting patient information and has confidence in his treatment of choice, the first consideration should be that possibly the patient is not following through with home applications of ice and Body Movements. If this is so, he should be reminded, again, of the importance of home treatments and that the progression from the Treatment of Pain Phase to the Corrective Phase is dependent on his participation. Patients who truly want to make this progression will be diligent in following instructions. There will, however, be a small percentage of the patient population that will continue to appear for treatments but will not participate in follow-through of any kind. These patients are usually deriving secondary gains from their condition and have either an emotional component or material compensation invested in their pain (see *The Low-Back Patient,* The Personality Profile of the Low-Back Patient, Chapter 1).

The patients who expect some type of material compensation for their pain/injury will continue to come for treatment for some time. They will report that although the original pain is somewhat improved, a secondary pain has replaced it and has become the object of the patient's pain focus. Their complaints will vacillate between those two areas.

On the other hand, a patient with an emotional investment in the pain will usually panic when it begins to disappear, and he will continue to display the same "unhealthy" outward behavior of limping, listing, having difficulty changing positions, etc., in an attempt to fulfill his dependent need for the love, attention and/or control of his family and friends. When this type of patient is confronted during treatment by therapists who are concerned with and reinforce only healthy attitudes and behavior, the conflict between what the patient needs for an unchanged environment and the behavior the therapist expects becomes too great and he will drop out early in the treatment program. The only hope for a patient of this kind is for his support group (family, friends, physician, etc.) to cooperate with the therapist in accepting and reinforcing only healthy behavior. Since most patients of this type are expert manipulators, close family and friends are often convinced that the patient is doomed to a life of pain and have adjusted their lives accordingly. Therefore, the therapist is confronted not only with an experienced "pain" patient, but a "conditioned" family and with a set of circumstances that cannot be altered until the patient decides that it is time for a change in his life status.

If the therapist decides, after taking into consideration the above possibilities (especially those of "secondary gain"), that the reports of pain are valid the treatment protocol should be altered. For example, he might choose to alter ice applications, i.e., to apply ice for a longer period of time or cover a larger area; to palpate for underlying triggerpoints; to give a direct application of electricity with a sound head; to recheck surrounding areas; or to suspect a more serious etiology or a chronic problem that may be reirritating the tissue. After checking further, the therapist would alter the treatment application in accordance with the needs of the newly discovered area(s) of abnormality. Pain will usually not disappear completely with one treatment (except when it is caused by simple muscle spasm from fatigue, overwork, etc.) but the therapist should expect the patient *to feel some change* in the area treated. In more serious conditions the patient should not expect all of his pain to disappear quickly or all at once, but he should expect constant changes in his body and condition, especially during the Corrective Phase of the therapeutic exercises. *Both the therapist and the patient should be constantly looking for subjective and objective changes in the patient's body as a result of the therapeutic treatment program.* Armed with this information of condition change, the therapist is able to properly motivate the patient and assist him in forming realistic expectations concerning the length of treatment and degree of relief he can hope to achieve. It is important to explain to the patient that even though some pain is still present, all evidences of *change* are important and are a positive sign that the patient's body is responding to the treatment. If therapy evokes the anticipated change in the patient's body, the treatment is correct and the patient is responding. If a patient has had pain for several years, it is unrealistic to expect it to disappear completely in a week or two of treatments, but the therapist will expect some significant change in the patient's condition. Sometimes the patient will feel the change although the therapist cannot always measure it. By the same token, the therapist may be able to measure a change but because of certain characteristics of pain and its perception plus a patient's psychological profile, the patient may not feel a change himself. At those times it is imperative for the therapist to point out the changes in the patient's body which occurred because of therapy. This will help to motivate the patient to continue with the therapy program and instill faith and hope for a successful outcome. If a change is not observed by either patient or therapist, the treatment is not effective and the protocol should be adjusted.

Success in the area of reassessment and program readjustment is predicated upon the fact that the therapist has assurance, confidence, and a high level of skill in the treatment he is delivering, which makes continuing professional growth on his part a necessity. Furthermore, if there is any question in the therapist's mind about whether a certain mode of treatment is best for the patient, he should definitely not be doing it. If there is another treatment that is more valid for a certain patient, it should be carried out. This may mean referring the patient to another medical practitioner or performing therapeutic techniques that take more time and effort. At all times, the needs of the patient must supersede those of the therapist. In other words, the therapist must be emotionally open at all times to the patient. This is sometimes more difficult than it sounds. All channels of communication must be kept open so that the therapist can receive all information possible. Everything about the patient's body must be learned, i.e., where ROM is limited; what soft tissue is lacking in flexibility; what area is restricted in function; where movement is not flowing properly; what alterations have taken place to the patient's general body posture; and where there is pain or emotional tightness. An article in *Brain/Mind Bulletin,* February 15, 1981, entitled "Neuro-K: Overcoming Disability with Sensory Awareness Training," states this necessity very well:

> "The "how to" of Neuro-K is unique to each patient. . . Often the therapist must intuitively know what needs to be done to accomplish the next step. This requires two simultaneous modes: 1) emotional openness to the patient; 2) analysis of every nuance of his physical movement. The patient must actively participate in learning. . . ."

While program reassessment and alteration is one important task of the therapist, another is patient education, which has many different areas and ramifications. The two main goals of this aspect of the Body Techniques program are: 1) to help the patient learn how to control his pain, and as a way of doing so, 2) to help him get more in touch with his own body. He must learn how his body responds to pain, to icing treatments, to movements, to exercises, to stretching, to tightness, and to loosening up again. There are going to be many changes in the patient's body and he has to come to terms with these changes because they often change him as a person as well. Patients usually become more open emotionally as their physical tightness and restriction disappears and most require the guidance of the therapist in both attaining the relief of pain and achieving body awareness and emotional health. The use of cryotherapy for pain control, breathing and relaxation for increased movement, and Body Movements to provide pain-free initial mobilization are three tools that the therapist uses to guide the patient. The patient's concentration of attention on his own body by comparing one side to another and by focusing on specific joint movements is also important. Each factor taken by itself may not seem all important, but together they produce a patient who knows his own body and can take the steps necessary to make it well. He becomes actively involved in his own therapy and remains active through the Corrective and Preventive Phases of treatment.

Subacute Stage

When the pain of muscle spasm has decreased substantially (which should be after two to five daily treatments in the office in addition to the patient's following through with ice and gentle Body Movements at home), he progresses to the subacute stage of the Treatment of Pain. By this time the therapist will have applied Body Techniques lightly but completely several times and will have discovered new areas of concentration. A restricted scapula, a sternocleidomastoideus that lacks flexibility and is not allowing proper movement, or triggerpoints in the cervical muscles are examples of what may have been identified. Whatever is the most immediate cause of the symptom of muscle spasm would be the area of concentration for the future treatments in the subacute stage.

A treatment concept that is important in both the acute and subacute stages of the Treatment of Pain therapy can be shown in the diagram below:

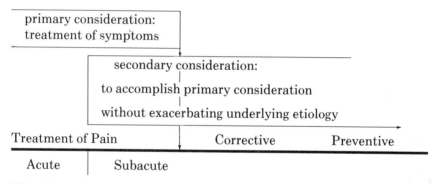

This chart illustrates that the treatment of pain is the first concern of the therapist in therapy BUT that it must always be done without causing an exacerbation of the underlying condition (secondary consideration), which is usually the more serious problem.

The treatment *components* most often used in the subacute stage of the Treatment of Pain Phase are:

1. Modalities
   A. low-volt electricity
   B. pulsed Ultrasound with electricity
   C. ice
2. Body Techniques (moderate applications with emphasis on areas of concentration)
3. Therapeutic Body Movements
4. Gentle therapeutic exercises

5. Home instruction
6. Education/Information

The *goal* of the subacute stage of therapy is treatment of the most immediate cause of the symptoms. In some cases the patient will skip this stage and treatment will progress directly to the Corrective Phase. Such a course would be recommended when all of the patient's pain disappears relatively quickly with treatment in the acute stage and does not reappear with functional activities. When this is the case, the underlying cause of the acute symptoms is usually identified through applications of Body Techniques and through further testing of the original area of concentration. The goal of the subacute stage of treatment is to eliminate the underlying cause of the muscle spasm and decrease any residual pain in this area. This will eventually allow the resumption of normal motion in the area of concentration. The patient should also be given therapeutic exercises to increase and maintain the newly acquired movement. If mild discomfort is felt while the exercises are performed or if the area is stiff or tight, the exercises could be done in the bathtub or shower where hot water will assist in loosening the area. If pain is more severe, ice (as carefully prescribed by the therapist) should be used on the area before exercising. Such preparation as is needed and the exercises themselves can be done one to three times a day depending on how intensely they affect the area. Of course, the patient should know why he is doing exercise and preparations, how they fit into the scheme of his treatment, and what the therapist expects they will accomplish. By making the patient a partner in the therapy, his strength and determination will be added to the therapist's own efforts to effect an improvement in the condition.

If an unusually stubborn triggerpoint (one cause of subacute pain) is identified during any treatment phase, combined *pulsed* Ultrasound and low-volt electricity would be applied repeatedly at subsequent treatments in conjunction with direct and deep acupressure and spray and stretch techniques to the muscle involved. Ice applications preceding the treatment will decrease the pain during acupressure. As soon as painless range of motion is achieved in the muscle and surrounding area, gentle stretching exercises preceded by heat should be introduced, and the patient should continue to perform them at home. Should pain be experienced during the stretch, ice should be reintroduced until movement can be achieved without pain. Subsequent treatments should be of low-volt electricity to the muscle involved (especially directed over the area of triggerpoint or restriction) to limber the involved muscles and to retain and encourage normal movement in the area.

Another cause of subacute pain is soft tissue restriction. Let us say that a patient had a muscle spasm in his cervical muscles and that it was treated in the acute stage. The therapist reduced the muscle spasm with ice, electricity, and Body Techniques. When the pain decreased, additional treatments of Body Techniques were given until the patient was pain free. No underlying causes (except perhaps a tight muscle) were found. The patient was given some stretches to do along with a few instructions on his posture. Everything else seemed to be in order and there was no underlying dysfunction. The pain did not return during functional activities, therefore, his problem was simply a soft tissue restriction, i.e., muscular problem in which there was not really any underlying joint problem. Normally, such a patient did not suffer from the pain for long periods and his pain was not the sequela of an earlier trauma. A patient of this kind would typically be having pain for the first time and it might have been due to some particular strain, postural imbalance, or sudden beginning of an unfamiliar activity or unilateral sport for which he wasn't conditioned.

Nerve interference is another cause of subacute pain. It normally occurs when there is a postural and/or mechanical imbalance that is causing pressure on a nerve. It takes about two months in the Corrective Phase of therapy to fully correct such an imbalance, but in the interim, the therapist must relieve the patient's pain. Once the muscle spasm is reduced, through the previously mentioned methods, the pressure usually remains and continues to reirritate the nerve until the area of concentration is mechanically "unloaded." Therefore, *the application of Body Techniques helps to relieve the pressure on the nerve temporarily until the patient is able to adjust his posture through a series of exercises which would be done in the Corrective Phase of treatment.*

Unequal weight distribution is sometimes the cause of subacute pain. A patient may be walking out of balance because chronically weakened muscles are ineffective in holding him upright against gravity. Sometimes he does so because of patterns induced by trauma. Suppose that he had a knee injury five years before and as a result has developed chronic weakness in that leg. The injury has caused him to put more weight on his unaffected side and that imbalance has caused pain in his low back because of strain. The acute stage of treatment would reduce the pain due to strain and muscle spasm and he would then move on to the Corrective Phase. Normally the therapist would use Body Techniques, along with other treatment modes that we have discussed to equalize muscular balance in the upper and lower back areas while isotonic or isokinetic exercises are prescribed for home use to strengthen the lower extremity, which would in turn help to improve general posture.

Finally, a symptom of habit which could cause a muscle spasm must be considered. If a patient holds a telephone to his right ear or holds a purse on her right shoulder continuously, chronic tightness in the right shoulder and right cervical area occurs. The area continues to be held in a shortened position, but not in spasm until the patient has an additional postural strain, emotional stress, or quick demand on the shortened muscles. The strain becomes too great and the muscle goes into spasm. While the underlying cause of the spasm is fairly simple and can be corrected with proper instruction, the pain must first be relieved before the patient will listen to advice on changing functional habits. The therapist must remember that *the most severe presenting symptom may not signal the most immediate underlying cause.* The same is true for less serious presenting symptoms. Therefore, the therapist must utilize palpation examination and functional testing to continuously search for additional causes of pain and dysfunction.

In summation: Four goals of the therapist in the treatment of acute and subacute pain *prior to* corrective therapy are:

1. relief of pain and promotion of pain-free movement
2. instilling faith and hope in the patient from the assurance, confidence, and skills of the therapist
3. education of the patient about his own body and his part in making it well again.
4. making it possible for the patient to perform the Corrective Phase of treatment with a minimum of discomfort

It is essential that the therapist assist the patient in performing the Corrective Phase of his therapy with a minimum of discomfort. No one wants to do corrective exercises when in a great deal of pain. It must be the goal of the therapist to substantially decrease or eliminate the pain (usually from muscle spasm and soft tissue distortion) in the acute and subacute stages to allow the patient swift progression into the Corrective Phase.

CORRECTIVE PHASE

Since the patient has progressed through the Treatment of Pain Phase in both its acute and subacute stages, he is now ready to enter the Corrective Phase. The goals of this phase of treatment are to identify (or substantiate the findings of the Initial Evaluation) and to treat (change) the underlying dysfunction causing the original pain.

There are two stages in the Corrective Phase of treatment: chronic and restorative. The chronic stage is so called to distinguish it from the most acute presenting symptoms for two reasons: 1) to underline the fact that the treatment must constantly change and that this change requires ongoing evaluation and reevaluation if the patient is to be permanently free from painful restrictions of function; and 2) to define chronic not as long-standing in terms of time but as a separate level of dysfunction requiring treatment of *specificity*.

The *treatment components* used most often in the Corrective Phase of treatment are:

1. All components used in the acute and subacute stages of the Treatment of Pain Phase
2. Flexibility exercises of specificity
3. Strengthening exercises of specificity (restorative stage)
4. Corrective exercises to be done independently by the patient at home which will reinforce the adjustments made in the office
5. Joint mobilization of specificity
6. Body Techniques (moderate to heavy applications)

Corrective exercises are given to increase movement of affected joints and restricted muscles until the patient reaches a mechanical balance in the area of concentration; pain-free function; normal (for the patient and condition) objective measurements; and *minimum* levels of strength necessary for support during daily activities.

The goal of the Corrective Phase of treatment is to identify and change conditions in the patient's body in order to accomplish a flow toward a more balanced state in every area (especially in the area of concentration). By constantly testing and comparing, therapist and patient can progress in the treatment so that the patient, in the restorative stage, will eventually reach his best possible pain-free, functional level.

It is important for the patient to be made aware of the fact that in the Corrective Phase of treatment there will be a heavier emphasis on therapeutic exercises. The patient will be expected to expend increased time and energy on his program as he will be performing more difficult exercises, including movements that may be painful and which usually will be preceded by either ice or heat. The patient will gradually assume more and more responsibility for his therapy. It is important at every step for the therapist to educate and support these efforts.

In the restorative stage of the Corrective Phase of therapy, exercises of specificity which increase the strength of the muscles in the area of concentration (using exercises which the patient can perform at home) are introduced. The goal of the restorative stage is to achieve an increased level of strength around a joint that currently has pain-free movement and flexible muscular components. This is most often done with cuff weights, pulleys, isometrics, or isokinetic exercises.

While most serious cases are treated in the Corrective Phase with both chronic and restorative therapies, some are not. In simpler cases, the patient may progress directly from the chronic stage to the Preventive Phase. Exercises of specificity or specific joint mobilization may be all that is needed. Each patient must be taken completely on an individual basis and each treatment tailored to his ailments and limitations.

Specificity

The two stages in the Corrective Phase of treatment—chronic and restorative therapy—usually work simultaneously. For instance, it is impossible to maintain the results of joint mobilization if the appropriate muscles are extremely tight, stiff, or weak. Therefore, the therapist begins to mobilize the joint, if need be, and at the same time prescribes the restorative, corrective exercises which are usually stretching exercises and exercises of specificity. "Specificity" is the important word here because the exercises prescribed are directed to the muscle or muscles which are preventing normal mechanical action in the area of concentration. They are picked specifically for the jobs that they do mechanically and because an increase in flexibility of the restricted muscles would allow for normal joint and area movement.

PREVENTIVE PHASE

When the area of concentration has full, or nearly full, function in terms of range of motion, flexibility, and minimum strength of individual muscles, the patient will progress to the Preventive Phase of therapy. Initially, the aim of this phase of treatment is to prevent future injury to the affected area until the patient learns how to use it normally again and incorporates its use into his daily activities. Toward this end, Body Techniques continue to be applied with moderate-to-heavy applications to return muscles to normal resting lengths repeatedly so that eventually they will maintain the new length independently without the tendency to remain shortened after use. Some patients develop triggerpoints or experience an occasional muscle spasm during functional use of a newly rehabilitated area. Body Techniques help to prevent these problems or, if they do occur, treat them. This allows the patient to progress to heavier strengthening and a higher level of functioning (such as sports) without feeling that he has had a setback or that even though he has been rehabilitated he has to "live with it" and still feels compromised.

In the restorative stage of the Corrective Phase of therapy, as soon as the patient gains minimum strength and normal flexibility around the joint, he can progress to conditioning exercises, such as Nautilus, Universal, Cybex, or more progressive PREs. In the Preventive Phase of therapy, he can add more functional kinds of strengthening activities to his program, such as bicycling, swimming, race walking, jogging, or whatever applies. Of course, the usual contraindications must be taken into consideration when advising a patient on any sport or functional activity. A patient with extensive arthritis of the spinal joints, even though pain-free after the therapy program, would not do well on a continuous year-in year-out jogging program, whereas he might do very well on a swimming program where there is no jarring or compression force on the joints. The original problem, how the patient got into his unhealthy state, and how the condition developed must all be considered when structuring functional activities for the patient's life after therapy. Further injury to the areas involved would be prevented by having him continue to perform conditioning exercises of specificity to the area of concentration. A variety of physical conditioning exercises would be prescribed in addition to an individualized therapeutic exercise program. Such a plan of treatment is an example of multisegmented therapy with ongoing assessment and treatment (see chart on page 78).

A patient who has been in considerable pain and who has progressed to pain-free function and prevention will, of course, have to maintain a program of physical conditioning indefinitely in order to prevent old troubles from recurring and new ones from appearing. It is an important part of the therapist's role to educate the patient in this respect. With the confidence and trust already established and the improvement that the patient can see in his own condition, he should be ready to assume a life-long program of conditioning. The therapist must define and devise that program for each individual patient and be available to each one if adjustments or encouragement are needed.

Shifting Responsibility

It cannot be stated too strongly that the general goal of Body Techniques in each phase of treatment is to return control of his own situation to the patient. At the beginning of each phase, the therapist assumes control of the therapy because he or she has the knowledge and skill to help the patient overcome that phase of the problem. The patient regains control when the teaching (by the therapist) and the learning (by the patient) is completed for the specific phase. This is another reason why education of the patient is so important and why the patient must remain active in the entire process. The passive personality is more apt to rely on drugs, surgery, or chiropractic treatment as solutions to his neck or back pain, as these treatments are more suitable to his emotional needs. The patient who presents his body for treatment to be cured in a passive way will probably not benefit completely from the approach used in the application of Body Techniques.

During the Treatment of Pain Phase and at the beginning of the Corrective Phase of therapy, the therapist is required to do most of the work and thus carries most of the responsibility for the success of the therapy. As the patient progresses further into the Corrective program, however, the responsibility shifts gradually. The patient continues to accept higher and higher levels of responsibility and to do most of the work independently. Finally, he must accept the responsibility for applying the individually structured program of uninterrupted exercises and conditioning that will keep him healthy during his lifetime.

SUMMARY

The Theory of Application is based on a structured, individually tailored, and progressive program. The *Initial Evaluation* provides information to both the therapist and the patient on the physical and personal aspects of the patient's problems. It makes possible an educated estimate on the therapist's part of the duration of the treatment schedule and what results can be realistically expected from it. The *Treatment of Pain Phase* is broken into acute and subacute stages during which the patient is relieved of debilitating pain. The *Corrective Phase* of therapy, in its chronic and restorative stages, seeks to restore pain-free function and normal movement to affected areas. The *Preventive Phase* reinforces the gains made in the area of structural change that the Corrective Phase began and works to keep the patient in the best, most functional state he can expect, given his particular physical condition.

While it is easy to summarize these stages of treatment, it is important to always keep in mind that the actual application of the treatment must be as varied and individual as each patient is different from all others. An infinite range and combination of therapies will be needed in treating many patients. Knowledge, confidence, experience, and the therapeutic touch will enable the therapist to adapt all treatment to his or her unique patient.

The goal of all treatment is, of course, to return the patient to full functional and enjoyable life within the limits of his general health status. It is implicit in this goal that the patient actively participate in his treatment and, finally, take complete charge of his own progress.

BODY TECHNIQUES THEORY OF APPLICATION

INITIAL EVALUATION: Communication; Rapport Building ↓ Amassing Evaluative Information
Establishing Levels of Treatment Priority
→
Patient Education

MULTISEGMENTED AND ONGOING ASSESSMENT AND TREATMENT:

Treatment of Pain Phase		Corrective Phase		Preventive Phase
Acute Stage: most painful acute presenting symptom	*Subacute Stage:* most immediate cause of symptom	*Chronic Stage:* underlying dysfunction	*Restorative Stage:* correction by exercises of specificity	*Maintenance:* maintaining gains by general conditioning exercises → recreational activities
Examples: • muscle spasm • inflamed or irritated soft tissue • fibrositis • pain due to poor posture or mechanical imbalances	Examples: • triggerpoints • soft tissue restriction • strain • nerve interference • unequal weight distribution • symptom of habit	Examples: • joint dysfunction • mechanical imbalances (i.e., pelvic obliquity) • contracted muscle • faulty posture • weakness • unequal weight distribution		
Levels of Responsibility (work required) during each phase of treatment: Passive for the patient; physical therapist does most of the work.		Patient regains 50% responsibility for therapy.		Patient takes 90% responsibility for therapy.

Chapter 4

Plan of Application

Each patient's comprehensive treatment plan is formulated by analyzing the results of the subjective report of the patient, the Initial Evaluation, and the therapeutic touch information gathered by the therapist during the application of Body Techniques. The treatment modalities which are available to be used initially are:

1. Breathing exercises
2. Relaxation training
3. Cryotherapy
4. Pulsed Ultrasound combined with electricity (subacute stage)
5. Electrotherapy
6. Gentle Body Movements
7. Body Techniques (light to moderate application)
8. Education/information
9. Positive reinforcement
10. Attitudinal formation

Modalities are never chosen randomly, to fill time, or for the convenience of the therapist. They are applied specifically to assist the therapist in achieving her goals for that particular treatment for the individual patient.

FORMULATING THE PLAN FOR TREATMENT OF PAIN

With a psychologically healthy patient, pain will most often be the entity that initially concerns us in formulating the plan and goal for individual treatments (Treatment of Pain Phase) while the dysfunction will direct us in the overall treatment protocol (Corrective Phase). For example, when a patient enters treatment because of a painful neck and shoulder on the right side, the subjective reports of pain interest us for two reasons. First, because the pain is of utmost importance to the patient and the primary reason that treatment is being sought. Second, because the complaints of pain are the first indication to the therapist of which structures are involved in the dysfunction and, therefore, define the starting point in the investigation of the underlying mechanical imbalances. If this patient happened to be in a career field which required a high level of physical performance or extensive periods in one posture (sitting or leaning over a desk), it would understandably be very upsetting if the therapist ignored or underemphasized the complaints of pain. The therapy would be inadequate if it merely treated the underlying physical structures involved while the patient's pain continued to cause limitation and undue suffering.

Therapists often make a mistake in attempting not to reinforce a patient's pain pattern by downplaying the importance of the reports of pain. This is indeed an error as, except with a very small number of patients who are receiving secondary gains from their pain (see the *Low-Back Patient*), each patient's pain level continues to be an indicator to the patient of how he is progressing in the treatment program. Pain or the lack of it determines to a large degree whether or not the patient will continue to have faith in the therapy or continue with the therapy at all. To the therapist, the patient's subjective pain reports are often indicators for selection of treatment techniques and of the patient's readiness for progression in the therapy. Therefore, the therapist must continue to be open to the reports of pain and use the information analytically in choosing treatment protocols. This is imperative in the Treatment of Pain Phase as no one knows where the patient's pain is being felt except the patient himself.

If the patient complains of pain in a muscle (subjective) which was in spasm when he initially came into treatment (Initial Evaluation) and the therapist palpated a triggerpoint (therapeutic touch) during a treatment, the treatment plan would then include the use of Ultrasound with electricity directed at dissolving the triggerpoint and the application of Body Techniques with a concentration on the area of the triggerpoint. To achieve lasting results, the patient would be required to follow through at home to reinforce the efforts of the therapist in dissolving the triggerpoint and also, in advanced stages of therapy, with corrective and preventive exercises to regain mechanical balance in the area of concentration if necessary. This multifaceted approach, with all efforts of the treatment (or several treatments), is required to achieve the desired result of a permanent pain-free status.

Muscle Spasm

Muscle spasm is usually the first entity to be treated. If the patient has suffered from an acute sprain, has developed a triggerpoint, or has a more serious etiology for his pain such as lumbar or cervical radiculopathy, the most painful presenting symptom will usually be muscle spasm. The *treatment plan* for a severe muscle spasm would be:

1. Ice packs or ice massage until the affected area is numb and painless
2. Application of electrotherapy to affected muscle group—five minutes tetanizing, fifteen minutes surge
3. Body Techniques—light application with concentration on acupressure and vibratory techniques
4. A second application of ice if necessary
5. Instructions for the patient to follow between treatments
6. Gentle Body Movements
7. Positions for the patient to avoid; proper positioning
8. Explanation of the patient's condition and reassurance that the treatment will reduce the pain

Deep breathing, as described in Chapter 2, is continually being emphasized during the application of Body Techniques.

Body Movements

The following gentle Body Movements are taught to the patient beginning at the first treatment. Controlled breathing and deep breathing methods are coordinated with the Movements and are an integral part of the exercise. Proper breathing is emphasized throughout, especially with patients experiencing high levels of pain or those who are tense or anxious.

"A simple breathing exercise enables people to alter short-term brain hemisphere dominance at will. The exercise has implications for voluntary control of body-mind states and suggests a link between Eastern and Western concepts of medicine.

"When airflow is more free in one nostril, the opposite hemisphere is currently dominant. Forceful breathing through the more congested nostril awakens the less-dominant hemisphere.

"The finding demonstrates the individual's ability to noninvasively, selectively, and predictably alter cerebral activity and associated physiologic processes." (David Shannahoff-Khalsa, *Brain-Mind Bulletin,* Salk Institute for Biological Studies, Jan. 3, 1983.)

Body Movements 1, 2, and 3 are taught to the patient at the end of the first treatment.

1. *The Head Wobble*
    The patient lies supine with a pillow under the knees. Standing at the head of the table, the therapist instructs the patient, "Let your

head fall to one side. Do not use any effort to bring it to the side, let it fall by itself. Use no effort to hold it in that position." The only effort in this exercise is in returning the head to the original position so that it is ready to fall to the other side. Once the patient has mastered letting go of the head, he is instructed to breathe into his stomach for as long as possible and to slowly let the air out through pursed lips as he lets the head fall. This exercise is more difficult than it seems and patients who are tense or in pain have difficulty in mastering it. If the patient does have difficulty letting go, the therapist can assist by rolling the patient's head to one side and adding a slight vibration of the head at the end of the range. This automatically relaxes all of the tense muscles in the neck.

2. *The Neck Push*

The patient remains in the same position and is instructed to inhale deeply. As he slowly exhales, he should push the back of his neck down into the table being careful not to let his rib cage raise off the table. This automatically causes the chin to move down into the neck which reverses the cervical lordosis. It also loosens the structures at the occiput and is the first proprioceptive exercise which teaches the patient the correct positioning of the head for proper posture, i.e., extension at the OA joint. The neck push is released when the exhalation is complete. The patient is encouraged to inhale/exhale for longer periods as time progresses so that he will be able to hold the push longer.

3. *Knees to Chest with Breathing*

The patient lies supine with no pillows. He brings one knee at a time up toward his chest and holds onto both knees with his hands. *He will not, at any time throughout the exercise, pull his knees to his chest.* He is instructed to let his arms be heavy as they hang onto his knees and breathe deeply into his stomach. As he begins to exhale, he will notice that his knees automatically move a little closer to his chest and the patient takes up the slack, which the breathing has created, by letting his arms become very heavy. After about a minute of breathing, he will find that his knees will be as close to his chest as they can get at this particular time in the therapy. The patient begins doing this exercise for one minute and gradually builds up to three minutes. Doing the exercise this way, as opposed to just pulling the knees to the chest, produces no strain to the area and does not aggravate the existing pain. Also, there is more movement between each vertebra rather than just pulling the pelvis forward as is the case when you grab your knees and pull them to your chest. Pulling your pelvis forward creates a strong pull on the lumbosacral area.

Utilizing the breathing technique for movement, as described in this exercise, prevents strain to the area, causes no reaggravation of pain, and induces movement between the vertebral segments.

At this point the patient is given a sheet of instructions for icing at home (see Chapter 3). He is instructed to ice the painful area first and then perform the Body Movements he has learned. This procedure is to be done twice a day and whenever the patient has pain. At the end of the second and third treatments, Body Movements 4, 5, and 6 are taught and added to the home regimen.

4. *The Pelvic Tilt*
  The patient bends his knees and puts the soles of his feet on the table. The therapist places her fingers under the patient's low back and requests him to: "Inhale/exhale slowly and, with concentration and control, push your low back down onto my fingers. Do not push with your feet. Use only your stomach muscles and pinch your buttocks together to achieve the push. Slowly let go." If the patient has difficulty in performing the tilt, have him arch the lumbar area first, then do the opposite, tilt downward. This position is held until the exhalation is finished.

5. *Neck Push and Pelvic Tilt*
  Both exercises are performed simultaneously while the patient exhales. The patient is told that he should feel the entire spine lengthen if he maintains the push in both the cervical and lumbar areas and if he pushes with enough effort and concentration.

6. *Neck Push, Pelvic Tilt, and Shoulder Wiggle*
  The Neck Push and Pelvic Tilt is performed while the patient exhales and, while holding this same position, loosens and wiggles the shoulders. This is done for two reasons: a) so that the patient will break the pattern of using his shoulder musculature to hold his head in an improper position in the sitting and standing positions; and b) to teach the patient proprioceptively where the different parts of his body should be during proper posture.
  This position of extended neck, relaxed shoulders, and tucked pelvis is learned and practiced in the supine position so that it will be carried over to the standing and other functional positions.

When most or all of a patient's pain has been eliminated, the Cat Back exercise can be added to the program.

Cat Back Exercise
  The patient is requested to get on his hands and knees with his hands underneath his shoulders. His elbows remain extended

throughout the movement. The therapist instructs him to "Raise your head up to look at the ceiling. As you do, slowly let the area between your shoulder blades go, let the mid-back go, and finally let the low back go." For obese patients or patients with exceptionally weak musculature in general, request that they maintain a slight abdominal contraction to protect the low back during the end of the arch. "Inhale deeply and slowly begin to exhale as you tuck your chin, round the shoulder area, then the lumbar area." Request that the patient use a final contraction of the abdominals at the end of the rounding to cause a further rounding of the low back. The object is to reach for the ceiling with the spine. The patient should continue to stretch the entire spine in this position even after the rounding position has been achieved initially. The therapist can assist by touching the different areas of the spine while requesting the patient to move or let go during both parts of the Movements.

Remember that the *goals* of the acute stage of the Treatment of Pain Phase are:

1. to eliminate or decrease pain
2. to release the spasm and tight muscles enough to examine underlying tissue and structures (through the application of Body Techniques)
3. to bring the patient to a point of decreased pain so that he will develop trust and faith in the therapist and in the program of treatment.

TREATMENT PROGRESSION

When the patient no longer requires cryotherapy at home between treatments and can perform all Body Movements with little or no pain, he is ready to do one of the following:

1. Progress to the subacute stage of the Treatment of Pain Phase for treatment of the most evident cause of the muscle spasm (trigger-point, restricted muscles, etc.) if it has not yet been corrected.
2. Progress to the Corrective Phase if the patient has more serious underlying mechanical imbalances which caused the original symptoms.
3. Be discharged pain-free and independent after the underlying cause for the initial episode has been uncovered (through applications of Body Techniques and traditional testing) and has been corrected.

Each patient when discharged should be provided with suggestions on proper posture (he has been given exercises to assist with this), how to avoid future aggravation of the area, its proper use, and the education received during therapy in the use of cryotherapy and Body Movements for future treatment should the muscle ever go into spasm again.

To illustrate these points of treatment progression, let us view the case histories of three patients.

Patient A is a secretary who leans over a desk and typewriter all day. She was fairly active and had no complaints other than a stiff, painful neck on the right side. She was confused because she had never had neck pain before although, on occasion, after playing tennis the right side of her neck would stiffen up. This occasional stiffness did not interfere with her work, however, the current neck pain did. Therefore, she was understandably concerned about performing at her job with normal efficiency.

During the Initial Evaluation, the patient was found to have intense muscle spasm in the right cervical musculature and severe pain with any movement of the head, neck, shoulder, or arm on the right side. There was no radiation into the right arm. She received the standard treatment for muscle spasm:

1. Ice packs
2. Electrotherapy
3. Light applications of Body Techniques with a concentration on acupressure and vibratory techniques to the affected area
4. Breathing exercises
5. Specific home instructions

She was instructed to avoid feeling any pain in the affected area, and whenever she did feel pain she was to stop what she was doing and apply ice until the pain disappeared. Only then was she to proceed to perform the Body Movements.

After receiving treatment for three days in succession, the spasm released. The patient returned the following week for two treatments and the spasm had not returned. Through the application of Body Techniques it was found that the right shoulder continued to be elevated; that there was tenderness at the right occiput; and also tenderness at the superior angle of the right scapula. The muscles remained tightened even after the spasm released. The two remaining treatments included heat, electrotherapy, Body Techniques, and flexibility exercises (subacute stage) for the affected area.

Since there was no remaining pain, Patient A was discharged with suggestions on how to maintain proper posture at her desk. She was also told how to avoid muscle spasm in the area by doing her Body Movements and flexibility exercises before and after playing tennis and whenever the muscles begin to tighten from postural strain or tension.

Patient B was referred by his neurologist with the diagnosis of cervical radiculopathy. He presented with pain on the right side of his neck with occasional radiation and tingling into the right arm and hand. The Initial Evaluation exposed a limited range of motion in the cervical area and right scapula and diminished reflexes in the biceps/triceps. There was also moderate spasm of the right cervical muscles.

In the acute stage of the Treatment of Pain, the patient received:

1. Ice
2. Electrotherapy
3. Body Techniques
4. Relaxation
5. Breathing exercises
6. Body Movements
7. Home instruction

He was treated three times a week and by the beginning of the second week the pain had subsided. At this point, during the application of Body Techniques, a painful triggerpoint was identified in the right trapezius muscle at the level C3-4. Pulsed Ultrasound combined with electricity was applied with a sound head held directly over the triggerpoint for several minutes. The muscle was then stroked with the sound head and several minutes of application was applied to the right occiput which was also tender and painful. (The patient can usually direct the therapist to the most painful points, and the sound head is held longer on these spots.) Ice, electricity, and Body Techniques were also applied. The patient followed up at home with ice, Body Movements, and a gentle lengthening exercise to the affected muscle.

After three treatments, the triggerpoint dissolved, the muscle was sufficiently returned to its resting length to prevent further spasm, and the patient was pain-free. During further evaluation, the patient was shown to be lacking in the end range of shoulder flexion and in scapular range of motion. In order to correct these limitations, Patient B was moved into the Corrective Phase of treatment. As the limitation was muscular, not skeletal, he received a stretching exercise to increase shoulder flexion and several treatments were given to mobilize the scapula in order to increase its range of motion. This goal was accomplished with treatments of Body Techniques and the addition of the traditional side-lying technique. A stretching exercise for the rhomboids and the middle trapezius muscles was taught to the patient so that he could maintain the results of individual treatments on a daily basis at home. During the week of mobilization treatments, there was a continuation of ice, electrotherapy, and Body Techniques to prevent further aggravation to the affected muscle.

After one month of treatment, Patient B was discharged pain-free with normal range of motion in the cervical, shoulder, and scapular areas. His posture had been corrected through the Body Movements, and he had learned that his trapezius muscles, especially the right, held most of his bodily tension during stressful periods or postural strain. His exercise program was tailored to rectify that tendency. He was also advised to avoid further spasm by preceding the exercises with applications of heat, if the muscles were just stiff or tight, or ice if any pain was present. His radiating pain had disappeared after the first week of treatment and had not returned.

Patient C had a more serious dysfunction. He had been plagued with a long-standing lumbar radiculopathy that had not responded to conventional treatments. The pain radiated to his right buttock and to the lateral aspect of the leg. His musculature was weak in general and his neck was stiff and in the forward head position. In part, the Initial Evaluation revealed the following Patient Profile:

Lacking in flexibility: Right hip flexor, rectus femoris, quadratus lumborum, cervical muscles, hamstrings bilateral, paraspinals and calves bilateral, 14 inches from the floor in forward flexion

Weakness: abdominals, left hip abductor, low back and buttock muscles

Structural abnormalities: pelvis elevated right side ¾ inch, rotated forward and to the left, lumbar and cervical segments lacking normal range of motion, forward head position

Patient's report of pain: neck (from time to time), low back, right buttock and leg, right groin. Pain increased with sitting, standing, driving for long periods. The patient first experienced this problem five years ago. He is 37 years old.

Previous treatment: had received traction in the hospital, analgesics, muscle relaxants, exercises, acupuncture, chiropractic treatment— all of which afforded only temporary relief.

TREATMENT OF PAIN PHASE

Patient C was given the standard treatment for minimal muscle spasm in the right low back. During this time he received Body Techniques which began to loosen his cervical, upper back, midback, and low back muscles. Initially, the electrotherapy was concentrated on the low back and buttock areas for pain relief. The patient found that using the ice at home and doing the Body Movements relieved the pain unless he did something specific to induce it such as sitting for too long, driving, etc. For a short period of time, all activities that caused a recurrence of the pain were eliminated from the patient's daily activities in order that the pain cycles that had developed over a long period would relax. This would also give the patient a pain-free period so that the therapy could progress to the Corrective Phase. Through the application of Body Techniques, several triggerpoints were identified and they received pulsed Ultrasound with electricity and were dissolved. The patient's neck and low back musculature began to loosen with the application of cervical Body Techniques and through the Body Movements. At the end of two weeks of treatment given four times a week, he felt generally better, experiencing pain only when he induced it. During each treatment session, whenever the movement was required, he was taught the proper manner in which to roll, turn, and get up and down from a chair, the floor, a bed, etc. He was given the transitional Cat Back exercise with no ill effects.

At this point, the goals of the Treatment of Pain Phase have been met and the therapist must decide into which treatment phase the patient will progress. Patient C has underlying mechanical imbalances which were determined during the Initial Evaluation; therefore, he will be placed in the Corrective Phase as we continue to follow him through his treatment program.

CORRECTIVE PHASE

The goal of the Corrective Phase is to correct the underlying mechanical imbalances that are causing the symptoms of pain and dysfunction. This usually involves a major change in structure to balance functional usage or to correct postural alignment. The following modalities are available to assist the therapist in this phase of treatment:

- All previous modalities listed under the Treatment of Pain
- Therapeutic exercises:
    flexibility exercises of specificity
    strengthening exercises of specificity
- Home exercises to reinforce the correction
- Joint mobilization/manipulation of specificity
- Body Techniques (moderate to heavy applications)

The pain control methods of ice, electrotherapy, and Body Techniques performed during the Treatment of Pain Phase are continued throughout the Corrective Phase because patients will not do corrective exercises if they experience an exacerbation of the pain. The patient interprets pain to mean either that the corrective exercises are making their condition worse, or that the therapy is not working to their benefit in general. It is especially important to continue pain control throughout treatment because, although the acute and subacute stages of pain have passed,the patient will not respond well to corrective therapy if he begins to experience a recurrence of pain no matter how mild it may be. To just teach a set of corrective exercises or to hand the patient a sheet of paper and have them do the prescribed exercises without utilizing the modalities of pain control would cause an increase in pain and would reinforce the idea in the patient's mind that physical therapy did not and will not work for them. No matter how effective the treatments have been as exhibited by objective measurements, if the patient continues to feel pain he will not proceed in the therapy because in his own mind, no matter how logical the explanations of the therapist, pain indicates that he is not getting better.

A vital principle in ascertaining the order of priority for the goals of the Corrective Phase of treatment is: *The symptom whose correction will have the least direct negative effect but still be crucial to regaining mechanical balance to the painful area is chosen for treatment first.*

In applying this principle to Patient C's treatment plan, the therapist will note that even though testing has revealed weak abdominal muscles, strengthening exercises for these muscles would put undue strain on the lumbar spine and thus would cause an exacerbation of the original pain. Vigorous stretching of the right rectus femoris and the iliopsoas would definitely help to mobilize the right hip and decrease future low-back pain by regaining the mechanical balance, but it would also cause excess arching of the lumbar vertebrae. Since the abdominal muscles are not strong enough to decrease and stabilize the lumbar lordosis, this excessive arching of the lumbar vertebrae would also cause pain exacerbation. Therefore, these types of exercises would be contraindicated at this point in the treatment plan. Direct and specific mobilization of the spine would not be appropriate at this time either as the stronger muscular imbalance must be corrected first if the mobilization is to have lasting effect and if the patient's posture is to be improved to a great enough degree to remove the negative mechanical forces from the low-back area.

Taking the above observations into account, the therapist would exclude any strengthening exercises at this time (they would merely strengthen and reinforce the existing mechanical imbalance), even though they are indicated as areas of concentration in the Initial Evaluation. Considerations such as these must be made continually during the initial stages of the Corrective Phase of treatment otherwise the patient's pain will be exacerbated by what the therapist thinks he "needs to do," and the patient will lose both faith in the treatment and trust in the therapist. This must be avoided at all cost.

A most important principle in this stage of the Corrective Phase is: *Prescribing strengthening exercises at the beginning of the Corrective Phase, when there are areas of concentration that lack normal flexibili-*

ty, is definitely contraindicated. Therefore, in reconsidering Patient C's
Initial Evaluation we would temporarily disregard the areas that indicate
weakness because we have decided that strengthening is not to be part of
this initial stage of treatment. We would turn our concentration to the
structural abnormalities and those areas which are lacking in flexibility.
The therapist's thinking could be structured as follows:

The cervical muscles and joints will be considered at this time because
it is important to get the patient's head and neck in the proper position.
This will remove some of the postural negative forces from the low back
and help to decrease the pain while not having a direct negative bearing
on the area. Hamstring flexibility could be considered next even though a
direct stretch of the hamstrings could have a slight negative effect by
tilting the pelvis or stretching the sciatica. To reap the benefits of the
stretch without incurring the negative effects,the therapist must think of
an indirect way to stretch these muscles. The paraspinals and lumbar and
thoracic joints have begun to be loosened mildly by the prescribed Body
Movements and also by application of Body Techniques. Because of this,
the patient has already progressed in the upper, middle, and lower back
to the point where he can feel the difference. The calf muscles have no
direct bearing on the back except for general posture, and since the
patient needs a good posture to stretch the calf muscles, the therapist
would postpone stretching of this area until later in the treatment.

Because Patient C's rectus femoris is tight in the anterior aspect of the
thigh and the hamstrings in the posterior aspect, and both influence the
position of the pelvis, the therapist would loosen these areas in an
indirect way through the use of:

Exercise 1: Hip Rolls
> The patient lies supine, with a pillow under his head, and is
> instructed to do hip rolls. With both legs extended, he rolls one leg
> inward as much as possible and then lets it roll back to external
> rotation. The effort is on internal rotation and the external rotation
> is accomplished by a letting go of the tightened muscles. He
> continues to do this exercise on each side for up to a minute and if
> the patient has no pain with that movement he can progress to
> internal rotation of both legs simultaneously.

This exercise accomplishes several things. It increases the range of
motion of the hip joint; stretches out the piriformis and other rotators of
the hip that are usually stiff and tight in patients with low-back pain; and
begins to loosen all of the muscles around the hip. Although this exercise
has an indirect bearing on the low back and a direct bearing upon the
surrounding muscles, it nevertheless does not exert a direct stretch.
Because of this indirect approach, a very gentle movement of the
hamstrings (which will begin to correct an area of concentration need) is

accomplished without increasing low-back pain. Now that the low back, buttock, and hip muscles have been activated, lengthened, and used normally through the therapeutic measures listed to this point (without an exacerbation of pain), Patient C can proceed to the following exercise.

Exercise 2. Hip Extension on Pillows

The patient lies supine with no pillow under his head and two pillows under his knees. He is instructed to "Inhale and while slowly exhaling, push the back of your knees down into the pillows until your ankles come up and your buttocks raise up from the table. While your buttocks are raised, give them an additional squeeze. Slowly let yourself down." *Note:* This exercise is contraindicated initially in patients who have spondylolisthesis and spondylolysis.

Since this patient has weak low-back muscles and his problem is in the lumbar area, we must refrain from heavy strengthening exercises at this time. We can, however, begin to get the involved areas *moving* again after a long period of inactivity induced by pain and interrupted nerve supply. This exercise accomplishes those goals and is also good for pain relief as it gets the gluteus muscles and the rotators contracting/relaxing again which will often relieve radicular pressure. Most patients with low-back pain find that these two *indirect* exercises allow them relief from pain and stiffness as the therapist begins to work on their areas of concentration.

Review of Patient C's therapeutic program during the chronic stage of the Corrective Phase indicates that:

1. He has been coming for treatment three times a week.
2. He has been receiving moderate application of Body Techniques
   a. to continue to keep the muscles healthy
   b. to encourage normal joint range of motion
   c. to release any triggerpoints that might have formed
   d. to release any muscle spasms before they have a chance to interrupt the therapy
   e. to continue to provide information that is needed regarding his body, condition, and exercises
3. He is receiving a continuous exercise instruction and review.
4. He is applying ice at home whenever he feels pain.
5. He is performing all of the exercises and the Body Movements twice daily. (His program is so short at this point that he is able to do it twice a day.)

The treatment will be decreased to two times a week as soon as the patient does not require ice for pain relief between treatments, knows his exercises well, and can perform them correctly.

As the patient continues to progress on this treatment program, the therapist must continually reassess the program and his patient's needs. Reassessment at this stage indicates that the demands that the Corrective Phase of therapy, Body Techniques, and home follow-up exercises have placed upon Patient C's body have begun to: loosen his cervical muscles; activate his abdominal muscles; and lengthen the paraspinals through the Cat Back exercise and forward flexion in Body Techniques. Now that he is free of pain, he is doing all of his Body Movements more vigorously, with increased control and exertion, and with normal contractions of the muscles. As a result these movements have become not only stretching exercises but mild strengthening ones as well.

As we review the Initial Evaluation list of concentration areas, we see that the therapeutic treatments given up to this point have begun to restore normal flexibility in Patient C's cervical and paraspinal muscles and he is beginning to develop some strength and control in the abdominal, low back, and buttock muscles. *There has been a great deal of progress made through the indirect approach without exacerbating the pain.*

Because the patient was able to tolerate the therapy without having to resort to the use of ice at home, the treatment can now proceed to a more direct and specific phase of correction. After reconsulting the patient's profile, the therapist would most likely decide to try the hamstring stretch. Prior to the actual stretch treatment, however, the modalities the patient is receiving would be adjusted in accordance with the patient's needs. If he has less than 60% of hamstring flexibility, the therapist would change the modalities preceding treatments to the following:

1. Ten minutes of electrotherapy—two electrodes on each side of the patient's low back for 10 minutes, to continue to keep that area healthy and loose; and using four pads on each leg (two pads to the quadricep, two pads to the hamstring) for ten minutes on a reciprocal setting, to duplicate the normal quadricep/hamstrings reciprocal action.
2. Ten minutes of heat—while the patient is receiving reciprocal electrotherapy on one leg, the assistant physical therapist is applying hot packs to the other leg. When the ten minutes is up, the electrotherapy is changed to the other leg and the hot pack is placed on the opposite hamstring.

The half-hour preceding the therapy would entail ten minutes of electrotherapy to the low back; ten minutes reciprocal electrotherapy to each leg; and alternating hot packs to each hamstring. The goal of this therapy is to keep the low-back musculature loose and flexible, to continue with pain control, and to assist the patient in loosening the hamstring muscles so that they are less painful while stretching. We accomplish this by the use of heat (which in itself adds 15% elasticity to the muscle) and electrotherapy. The patient is now ready for:

Exercise 3: Hamstring Stretch

The patient lies supine with no pillow under the head. The knees are bent and the soles of the feet are on the floor. The commands of the therapist are: "Bring your knee up toward your chest. Bend your ankle up. Inhale and as you slowly exhale, straighten your leg until you can lock your knee." The patient brings his leg as high as possible without bending his knee. The object of this exercise is to keep the knee locked at all times and to bring the leg up as high as possible. When the patient brings his leg up and locks his knee he is not doing the exercise, he is merely assuming the position. The exercise itself begins when the patient inhales/exhales as he continues to lock the knee and at the same time raises the leg as high as possible while keeping the ankle dorsi-flexed.

This is a good beginning stretch. After the patient can perform this exercise for a week or so with no exacerbation of pain, he is then ready for a progression.

Exercise 4: Hamstring Stretch Progression

The patient lies supine and assumes the position in Exercise 3. With knee locked, leg extended upward, the patient tucks his chin and reaches above the knee joint with the fingers of both hands. As he inhales/exhales, he brings his arms toward his body by flexing his elbows while pushing his locked knee away in the opposite direction. This gives a maximum stretch, especially to the distal aspect.

The patient is instructed to continue these hamstring stretches at home and is also informed of the fact that if he precedes his stretching with a hot bath that the heat will greatly enhance the stretching capabilities and will also reduce the discomfort of the stretch. The breathing is very important in the stretching exercises for the alleviation of this discomfort. It would be helpful to the patient if he were made aware initially of the fact that there are certain muscles which are very painful when they are being stretched. The hamstrings and the quadraceps group are two of these muscle groups which are painful when being stretched effectively.

As noted previously, correct breathing is very important in the exercises because:

1. It enables the patient to experience as little pain with the stretching exercises as possible
2. It helps the patient to avoid straining (Valsalva's effect)
3. It encourages mind/body coordination during exercise

This is another reinforcement of the principle that *every method is utilized that can reduce the pain that the patient experiences while doing the exercises.*

At this point in the treatment program. Patient C's subjective reports are enthusiastic. He is feeling better than he has in years. His neck muscles are loose and he has no more neck pain. It is easier for him to reverse the forward head position because the therapist has been adjusting him in that position with every Body Techniques treatment and has been loosening all of the structures that have been preventing him from maintaining that position. He has gained minimal strength in his stomach and low-back muscles through Body Movements and by having been previously advised to hold in his stomach muscles at all times. He is aware also that this stomach control will activate the buttock muscles and will tilt the pelvis. Through being coached on proper movements throughout each treatment session, he has virtually gained more control over his body and returns to treatment with a good posture, a loose back, freedom from pain, and an optimistic psychological outlook. Patient C feels at this point that he has achieved another level of health and realizes that he is working on the underlying conditions which caused his pain. He is now ready to proceed to a more specific and restorative stage in the Corrective Phase of treatment because:

1. He requires no applications of ice at home, because he is free from pain (he reports discomfort in the hamstrings during stretching, which is to be expected, but no pain reported in the back).
2. He has been motivated and educated all along the way and is therefore able to treat slight pain at home, should it occur, with the proper applications of ice/heat.
3. He is actively participating in his exercise program because he is aware of the progress being made and the rationale of the treatment in general.

The therapist will now add to Patient C's treatment program a stretch to begin to loosen the right rectus femoris since the tightness of this muscle is limiting the proper positioning of the patient's pelvis.

Exercise 5: Rectus Femoris Stretch (Figures 1, 2, and 3)

The patient is asked to come to the edge of the plinthe. He is on his back at the edge of the plinthe with his right side toward the edge. He is asked to drop his right leg off the table and to hold his right ankle with his right hand. If the rectus femoris is very tight, the patient will be unable to accomplish this movement. The therapist will then assist the patient by placing his or her right hand upon his right knee and will hold that stable. The therapist will then ask the

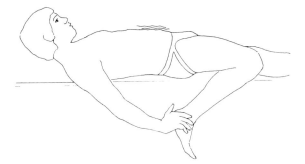

Figure 1

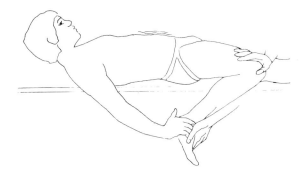

Figure 2

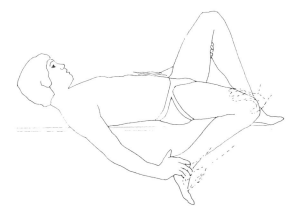

Figure 3

patient to inhale and, while he slowly exhales, to bring his head up and pull in his stomach. This will stabilize his low back to the plinthe to protect his lumbar vertebrae. If his muscles are still too weak to accomplish this, he can use his left hand to hold onto the opposite edge of the plinthe or to his left leg for support.

While the patient continues to inhale/exhale, the therapist slightly increases the pressure with her right hand to his right knee and uses her left hand on his right ankle to increase knee flexion and hip extension. This produces a major stretch on the quadriceps and especially the rectus femoris. This is held to the patient's tolerance for as long as possible while he continues with proper breathing.

For the patient who is not as severely limited and also for the above mentioned patient who progresses through treatment to a lesser degree of limitation, there will be no need for the assistance of the therapist during the exercise. The patient will be able to reach down to hold onto his own right ankle with his right hand, which will in and by itself place a stretch upon the quadriceps.

As he inhales/exhales, brings his head up, tucks his chin, pins his low back, and continues to increase knee flexion and hip extension, he will be placing a direct stretch on the rectus femoris. He must protect the lumbar vertebrae by pinning his low back to the plinthe. This is done by bringing up the head, pulling in the stomach muscles, and, if necessary, using his left hand on the edge of the plinthe or on his left leg for stability.

A *recap* of Patient C's total program indicates that at this point in the treatment scheme he is receiving treatment two times a week. This treatment encompasses Body Movements, Exercises, Hamstring Stretches, Rectus Femoris Stretches, and Body Techniques with no pain. He is also continuing his home exercise program twice a day. If the patient presents with pain symptomology at this stage in his program, the therapist must become a detective. The first assumption would be that the patient is not doing something correctly in one of his therapeutic exercises. He would be asked to show exactly what he is doing at home, how he is doing the exercise, and when the pain occurs in the movement. In so doing, the therapist should be able to pinpoint the area of incorrect application, and the correction of such should eradicate the pain. It is very unusual for the pain to recur in its original presentation in the low back at this point in the treatment program. If it does it is usually brought about by an overextension of muscle use, such as shopping in high heels for a woman or driving or sitting in one position for five or six hours. Patient C, because of the education he has received, is able to handle pain of this nature with the correct application of ice and corrective exercises. He no longer reacts to such pain with frustration or despair because he has learned the proper techniques of self-treatment. He is also confident that he can report his experience to the therapist at his next treatment and together they will logically overcome any obstacles to proceeding with the therapy.

Now that Patient C has achieved a minimal amount of flexibility in the quadriceps and the rectus femoris specifically and has more postural control, he is ready to add three new exercises to his home therapy program. These exercises will stretch the quadratus lumborum and are the most specific exercises that have been introduced up to this time because they are directed to the area that affects the muscles which actually attach to the lumbar vertebrae. When these exercises are taught to the patient, it is desirable for him to feel the stretching discomfort in the muscle that is being stretched but not to the point of feeling any radiating pain. At this point, the patient would be expected to be able to do the exercises correctly without inducing the original pain although he would feel stretching discomfort in that area. He must be taught to feel the difference as he learns the exercises.

Exercise 6: Pelvic Tilt with Rotation Against the Wall (Figures 4, 5, and 6)

The patient stands about 12 inches away from the wall; feet shoulder length apart; knees bent. He puts his low back against the wall up to his shoulder blades (the whole area between pelvis and shoulder blade is touching the wall). Shoulders are relaxed and head is in the proper position. The patient must pull in his stomach, pinch in his buttock muscles, and push with his feet to get a very strong contact of his low back against the wall. He should not use his shoulder muscles to accomplish this. When he has a very good contact, the therapist advises him to rotate slightly to the left so that one arm is on each side of his left leg. The patient tucks in his chin, pulls in his stomach, and hangs over his left leg. During this entire time he is using his abdominal muscles to strongly push the low back against the wall, especially on the right side. The therapist must constantly coach him to do this. A very strong stretching discomfort on the right side should be felt, and if it isn't, the patient will know that the exercise is being done incorrectly. In order to come up from this position, the patient should pull in his stomach until he comes up as far as possible and then rotate back to the center, so that he is not doing a flexion-rotation exercise while returning to the upright position. He will then proceed to do this same exercise on the left side with some stretching discomfort but not of the same intensity as the discomfort on the right side.

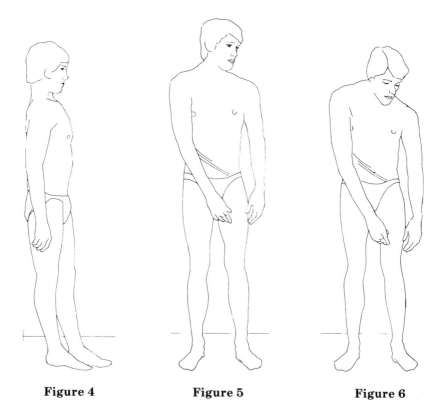

Figure 4   **Figure 5**   **Figure 6**

The goal of this exercise is to equalize both sides so that the right side, when he does the stretch, feels the same as the left side. This type of exercise is very convincing to the patient in showing him that the discrepancy is on the right side and that this exercise will help him to eventually even out the imbalance. Keep in mind that the patient is still receiving electrotherapeutic loosening of the quadratus lumborum area enabling him to perform the exercise without causing the original symptoms. Our continuous goal of increasing the exercise program without causing pain is being met.

After practicing this exercise, along with the others previously prescribed, at home for a week, he is ready for the addition of the needed calf stretch. The patient is ready for this because he has regained a good posture and has more control over each individual part of his body. He can do this exercise now without increasing his lumbar lordosis; without having a forward head position; and without putting stress on his back.

Exercise 7: Calf Stretch Against the Wall

The patient stands an arm's length away from the wall with his heels pinned to the floor. The palms of his hands are placed on the wall. His body remains straight as he drops from his hands to his forearms on the wall. He inhales/exhales; leans more onto his forearms; back straight; pelvis tucked under; heels pinned to the floor. After he holds this position for several inhalations/exhalations (which is about a minute), he puts his left leg forward onto his toes while bending the right knee of the leg that he is standing on in order to stretch the deeper calf muscles (soleus).

In reviewing at this stage the Patient Profile–Lacking in Flexibility, we find that the patient has been provided with a stretch for the hip flexors (the iliopsoas); the rectus femoris; and the quadratus lumborum. The cervical muscles have been worked on and stretched by Body Techniques, and the hamstrings are being stretched actively through therapeutic exercises. The paraspinals are being stretched in Body Techniques and the calves are being stretched by the last exercise given to the patient. As noted in the Patient Profile, Patient C was initially evaluated as being 14 inches from the floor in forward flexion. Being aware of the fact that there are two major muscle groups that restrict a patient in forward flexion, i.e., the hamstrings and the paraspinals, the therapist has prescribed individual stretching or flexibility exercises for each of these muscles. There will be additional motivation for the patient when he is retested on forward flexion at this time and finds himself to be only six inches from the floor. This is a vivid illustration of the gains made in a *functional* area. In other words, Patient C is now able to see that the treatments, hard work, and self-discipline have combined with the therapist's expertise and produced a functional gain which is enabling him to accomplish his goals in his daily activities.

Returning to the Patient Profile–Weakness, we see that the treatment program has indirectly affected the low back and abdominal muscles, but has not yet included an exercise for the left hip abductor because up to this time a PRE for the muscle would have aggravated the original area of concentration.

Comparing Patient C's present situation to his original Patient Profile–Structural Abnormalities, the pelvis is still elevated on the right side and is rotated to the left (none of the major skeletal work has been attempted yet). The lumbar and cervical segments that were lacking in normal range of motion have been somewhat affected in a direct way through the application of Body Techniques and indirectly by the therapeutic flexibility exercises. The forward head position is decreasing as time goes on through Body Techniques, postural training, and patient application of treatment concepts during functional activities.

If we look at Patient Profile–Report of Pain, we see that this patient has no neck pain, no low-back pain, no pain to the right buttock, leg, or groin. If any pain does occur during this period, it is that which comes from postural strain, i.e., holding a position for two or three hours, or from the patient incorrectly applying one of the therapeutic exercises.

Psychologically, Patient C has changed from a pain-racked individual, totally frustrated by the inability of the disciplines previously consulted to ease his pain and conquer his problem, to a pain-free person with trust in his present treatment, faith in his therapist, and confidence in his ability—through the education he has received—to control his own life again. Needless to say, we have on our hands a very pleased and motivated patient and also a therapist who can rest in the knowledge that his time and efforts were spent in a professional area of need and satisfaction.

Now that the patient has reached this point, we are for the first time going to consider treating the major structural changes indicated in Patient Profile–Structural Abnormalities. This area of patient treatment concentration is able to be considered at this stage in the treatment program because:

1. The muscles are pain-free and at their resting length.
2. The triggerpoints have been dissolved.
3. The muscle spasms have been reduced.
4. Pain is under the patient's control.
5. The muscles are working at minimum efficiency.

Since Patient C's profile indicates that the pelvis is elevated on the right side and rotated to the left, the first structural change to be made is in the area of pelvic elevation. The following exercise is a preliminary one that will assist in accomplishing that goal.

Exercise 8: Standing Side-Bend (Figures 7 and 8)

The patient intertwines the fingers of both hands. He turns the palms upward; inhales deeply until the elbows are completely extended; and stretches so high toward the ceiling that he feels the pull of the abdominal muscles on the pelvis. He then begins to slowly exhale as he bends to the left side. The patient tries to keep his pelvis level by maintaining normal and equal weight on the right and left foot. All of the stretch comes from the pelvis above. The patient leans over to the left and drops his head onto his left elbow. Continuing to inhale deeply/exhale, he goes all the way to the left side, being careful to extend the elbows and to reach outward as he

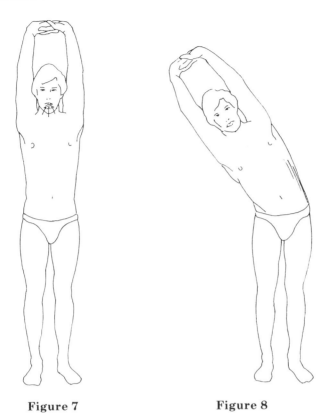

Figure 7   **Figure 8**

does so. He holds this position for three to four deep breaths. It is very important for the weight distribution to be evenly divided on both feet. Patient C would feel a much greater stretch on the right side as opposed to the left because his pelvis is elevated on the right and all of the attaching musculature is tight.

As he leans to the left, the muscle tightness on the right will cause his rib cage and axilla to rotate toward the left. When this happens, a great part of the stretch is lost because the tight muscles on the right side are not receiving a maximum stretch. In order to counteract this, the patient should take extra care to retract his right shoulder and derotate his rib cage toward the rear. If done correctly, this exercise will treat the very deep muscles that are reinforcing the elevation of the pelvis and rotation of the rib cage.

The exercise (another of those which allows the patient to experience the limitations of one side as opposed to the other) is to be repeated three times on each side with a concentration on position and deep breathing. The patient's goal is to create equal flexibility on both sides. This should take about two weeks to accomplish.

Now that we have begun to treat the pelvic elevation problem of Patient C we will attend to the rotational aspect. This rotational problem is due to tightness in the quadratus lumborum and paraspinals; the left hip abductors; and of the abdominal muscles on the right side. Restricted motion of these muscles on the right side will rotate the pelvis to the left anterior and the rib cage to the right posterior.

After the patient has been executing the standing side bend for two weeks, has no exacerbation of pain, and begins to feel relief from the right side stretch, he can be started on a Roman Chair routine as a progression. The Roman Chair is a piece of standard gym equipment which allows the patient to do complete side bending with the addition of his body weight in the direction of gravity. In this manner, we can accomplish maximum stretching of lateral trunk muscles including the abdominal and the oblique abdominal muscles.

Exercise 9: Roman Chair #1

The patient hooks his ankles at the left corner of the Roman Chair. Keeping his body straight but at an angle to the Roman Chair, he puts his left hand down on the floor and begins with deep breathing to let the top part of his body stretch (see Figure 9). The stretch will

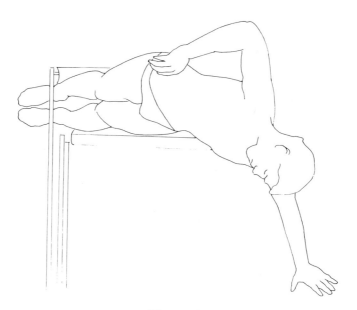

Figure 9

be felt along the tight areas of the right lateral trunk muscles. As he breathes into the stretch he begins to let his left elbow flex or bend so that his body weight and his head will go closer to the floor (see Figure 10). He continues with deep breathing until he feels a very deep stretch on the inside of his pelvis on the right side, and while continuing the deep breathing raises his right arm overhead (see Figure 11) and holds that position to tolerance. He then puts his right hand on the side of his pelvis and uses those muscles to pull himself up (see Figure 12). This exercise will also be repeated on the left, and the patient will see a vast difference between the sides, with a great deal more stretching discomfort on the right side as opposed to the left.

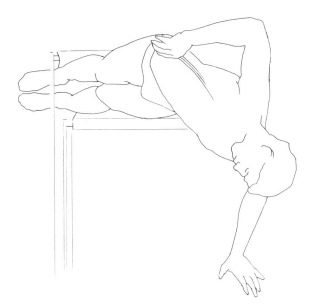

Figure 10

Patient C could complete his treatment with Roman Chair routine #1 by doing twice as many stretches on the right side as on the left. This is indicated because the right is the side that he is limited on and also the side of abnormal pelvic elevation. If he were going to do four pelvic stretches on the right he would do two on the left or if he were going to do one on the left he would do two on the right. The goal of this routine is to equalize the two sides so that he would feel the same on the right as on the left. After Patient C was doing this exercise for a week or two a progression would be added.

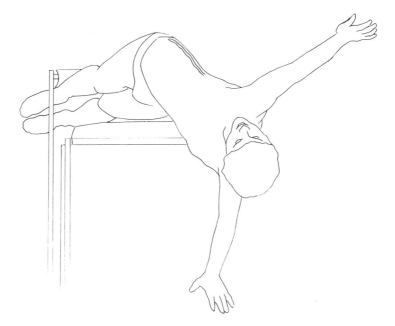

Figure 11

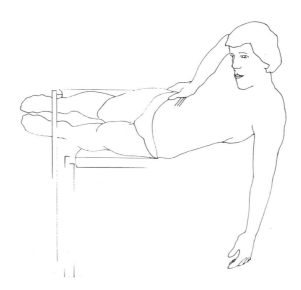

Figure 12

Exercise 10. Roman Chair #2

The patient assumes the original stretch position on his right side with his right hand on the floor and his right side pointing to the ceiling. While breathing and relaxing, he gets a maximum stretch on the right pelvic muscles and then rotates his body forward to the right by reaching through to hold the leg of the chair which produces a stretch on the posterior back muscles (see Figure 13). He breathes into this stretch and releases all of the tightness. He comes back to neutral and then rotates his rib cage to the rear as he did in the side bend. In so doing he will release all of the tightness in the right abdominal muscles. The same principle of doing twice as many on the right as on the left holds true but always only to the patient's tolerance.

The Roman Chair routines cause deep stretching of muscles and stimulation to joints, thereby assisting in loosening the structural abnormalities, which in Patient C are the pelvic elevation and pelvic rotation. The left hip abductor in Patient C also needs to be strengthened. Therefore, after the patient has executed the Roman Chair routine for one week without exacerbation of pain, the therapist will add a PRE with appropriate weight to the left Side-Bend routine. This is an exercise of specificity for strengthening the left hip abductor and will be given in both fast and slow components.

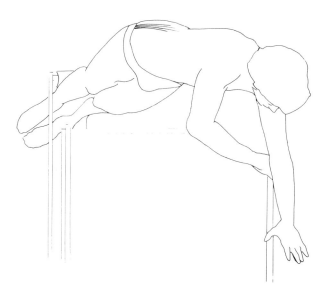

Figure 13

Progressing through the final stages of the Corrective Phase, the use of the Roman Chair routines places Patient C in the restorative stage making rapid progress toward the Preventive Phase. At this time he is fairly independent but is still unable to participate in any other physical activity such as tennis, swimming, jogging, etc. He will continue to be so limited until he enters the Preventive Phase of treatment. The twice a week treatment schedule will be reduced to once a week after he learns and masters the Roman Chair routines. His ability to function in his lifestyle has increased and he now reports being able to sit and stand for extended periods of time as well as realizing progression in all of those dimensions which originally had been a source of pain or limitation during ADL activity.

PREVENTIVE PHASE

Once the patient has been on the Roman Chair routines for two weeks, he will feel much better and will be asking about returning to other activities in which he had been participating before his pain caused him to seek therapeutic treatment. The therapist should give guidance at this time by instructing the patient in the gradual addition of activities such as swimming, walking, race walking, or a Nautilus conditioning program. The patient chooses one of these programs to augment his therapy. As he returns once a week for therapy, he will progress into the Preventive Phase of treatment by learning whatever specific PRE or conditioning exercises he requires. He will also be taught a straight back Sit Up/Sit Back exercise, first on a mat with later progression to execution on the Roman Chair.

Exercise 11: Sit Up/Sit Back (Figure 14)
    The patient sits on the plinthe with his knees bent and the therapist holding down his feet. He assures the correct posture by assuming the "Neck Push" position, arching his back normally, and keeping his spine very straight. His hands are placed on his knees or are crossed on his chest. The exercise consists of sitting back in three different positions. The first position is attained by coming back approximately one fourth of the way down and holding to the count of six while exhaling. Position two is another fourth of the way; hold for six; exhale. Position three is just several inches from the plinthe; hold for six seconds; exhale.
    If the patient has a great amount of weakness, he will just barely be able to accomplish this. However, if he has only moderate weakness, he will be able to finish the exercise by coming back up, slowly returning through the positions he took on the way down. In

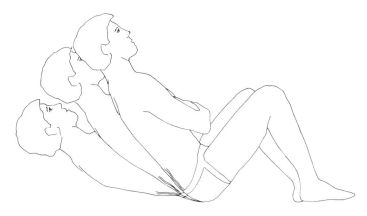

Figure 14

> other words, position three on the way down becomes position one on the way up.

This exercise not only strengthens the abdominal muscles but also strenghtens all of the postural muscles that the patient needs to retain good posture during functional activities. Because the traditional sit up strengthens the muscles that usually reinforce the posture of forward head, protracted shoulders, and thoracic slump, it is therefore not indicated as effective treatment for this patient.

The Preventive Phase is a culmination of the therapy program. All previous treatments have been building toward the climax of Patient C's program. Since the beginning of treatment, we have been educating the patient in the proper posture and prescribing exercises and Body Movements to achieve this desired state. We have treated his pain and even more importantly have taught him how to handle it should it ever return. Our patient's pelvis has been almost totally straightened and will be equal after he has worked out on the Roman Chair for a month or two. He knows the stretches to do if his side gets tight (Standing Side-Bend at home or stretch out in the gym). He has returned to light activity such as swimming or a progressive Nautilus program. We have eliminated his medical problems—pain and structural abnormalities—and have brought him up to a minimal level of strengthening through the use of therapeutic exercises and Roman Chair routines and have also taught him correct posture so he is now able to begin his activities like swimming or Nautilus. When he has been on those programs for two or three months with no exacerbation of pain—visiting our office every two weeks—he will be able to go on to other areas of activity such as jogging. Although jogging is not recommended for patients with serious postural, neck, or back problems, a patient who is young, healthy, and strong can gradually edge back into that routine if he or she wishes.

In summary, the Preventive Phase is the shortest phase of treatment due to the fact that we have been working up to it throughout our treatment program. The patient becomes a lot more independent at this stage because: he is feeling better; he has no pain; he has been educated; and he continues to receive guidance. The therapist has an opportunity at this time to introduce any other therapy that might be indicated for a particular patient. For example, if the patient has protracted shoulders from being in the forward head position for a long time, several exercises to reverse that condition might be added. One such might be:

Exercise 12: Pectoral Stretch in the Doorway
This exercise is done by the patient standing in the middle of the doorway with his hands extending backwards on the doorjamb. He walks straight through the door with his hands holding onto the doorframe. He continues to walk through until he stretches out his pectoral muscles and the shoulder joints.

Different types of postural exercises such as this can be added to the therapeutic program in the Preventive Phase.

Patient C at this point no longer feels like a patient. He has had a complete eradication of pain, his structural abnormalities have been changed, and his flexibility is in the normal range of motion. He has resumed his familiar activities and lifestyle and is completely satisfied with the therapeutic program he has received.

This program—which has been followed in detail in this chapter—is an example of the multifaceted treatment approach called Body Techniques. It must be stressed again that Patient C's program is individualized and is in no way to be construed as "the treatment" for all patients with similar symptomology. There is no standard treatment plan because Body Techniques treats *individuals* in an *individualized* program.

SUMMARY

The Plan of Application for each individual patient is arrived at by combining the knowledge acquired through the subjective report of the patient, the Initial Evaluation, and the therapeutic touch information gathered by the therapist through the application of Body Techniques. It consists of three Phases—the Treatment of Pain Phase in its acute and subacute stages, the Corrective Phase in its chronic and restorative stages, and the Preventive Phase. Each Phase has its own general goal with the addition of particular treatment goals structured to meet the needs of individual patients. There is a carry-through of one phase to the next in a continuously building process culminating in the accomplishment of the ultimate goal which is the resumption of normal daily activity.

During each of the phases, the modalities of ice, heat, pulsed Ultrasound, and electrotherapy (individually or in combination) are applied to the area of concentration and are combined with Body Techniques in order to relieve pain or prevent exacerbation of pain during the exercises. Patient follow-through at home is a vital part of the program because the efforts of the therapist in reducing muscle spasm, dissolving triggerpoints, or regaining mechanical balance must be reinforced for a successful final result. The continuous education of the patient is also an essential facet of therapy since the ultimate goal is for the patient to be aware of all of his body structure and musculature and to be able to handle minor symptoms of pain and tightness as he resumes his normal lifestyle.

The first and foremost area in the Plan of Application is the Treatment of Pain Phase. Its goal is the elimination of presenting pain in the acute and subacute stages as well as the individual patient goal of pain relief prior to and during the other phases of the program. This continual emphasis on pain relief or control carries throughout the entire Plan of Application for each patient and is accomplished by proper use of modalities, deep and controlled breathing, Body Techniques (as described in Chapter 2), and Body Movements (as described in Chapter 4). When the goals of the Treatment of Pain Phase (see page 59) have been reached, the patient is ready to be discharged or to proceed to the Corrective Phase of therapy.

During the Corrective Phase, the therapist continues previous pain control modalities, Body Techniques, and Body Movements while beginning in a logical and organized manner to treat each area of structural abnormality discovered during the Initial Evaluation. The Plan of Application in the Corrective Phase is based totally on the principle that the symptom whose correction will have the least direct negative effect but still be crucial to regaining mechanical balance to the painful area is chosen for treatment first. Strengthening exercises at the initial level of the Corrective Phase are contraindicated because they will create too great a strain on the area of concentration and will merely reinforce existing mechanical imbalances rather than correct them. Direct and specific mobilization of the spine in the initial stages of the Corrective Phase is also inappropriate because the muscular imbalance must be corrected first if the mobilization is to have lasting effect and if the patient's posture is to be improved to a great enough degree to remove the negative mechanical forces which often exacerbate the original pain.

Keeping the above principles in mind, the therapeutic program in the initial stages of the Corrective Phase consists of exercises which accomplish structural change and cause an increase in flexibility through *indirect* means. When these goals have been reached with no exacerbation of pain, more direct and specific exercises are added to the program. When a patient's muscles are pain-free, at their resting length, and working at minimum efficiency, the major structural abnormalities which are listed in the Patient Profile can be treated. At this point, the Roman Chair routines are introduced for deep stretching of all lateral trunk muscles and this marks the beginning of the restorative stage of the Corrective Phase of treatment.

The restorative stage includes the Roman Chair routines for deep muscle stretching and joint stimulation with the addition of PRE's for specificity. It also sees the introduction of the straight back Sit Up/Sit Back Exercise to strengthen abdominals and trunk muscles and to reinforce correct posture. This marks the end of the restorative stage and leads the patient into the Preventive Phase. It is at this time that the activities which the patient had previously enjoyed such as swimming, race walking, jogging, Nautilus, etc., may be resumed with a gradual building to full participation.

If the therapist has effectively evaluated the patient's therapeutic needs, treated the areas of concentration, altered structural abnormalities, strengthened areas of weakness, suggested physical activities which can be resumed, and, most importantly, educated the patient to all of the aspects of his individual program, recovery should be complete. This goal of complete resumption of pre-problem activity will be reached if each phase of treatment is applied correctly and continued until the goal of that particular phase has been attained. The Plan of Application is just that: a plan which is thoroughly investigated, structured, individualized, and then followed to a conclusion of maximum effectiveness with room for alterations as dictated by patient need. It should produce a "normal" functioning human being capable of returning to previous activity and lifestyle modes.

Chapter 5

Practical Applications
in a Clinical Setting

The Body Techniques program is flexible in application. A patient can begin treatment at any stage on the continuum and progress with ease within the treatment scheme at whatever pace necessary for complete recovery. The condition of the patient at the time of treatment coupled with the professional judgment of the therapist are the factors which decide the protocol for each specific treatment. Because the treatment plan is continually changing to parallel the condition of the patient, the therapist's judgment in applying Body Techniques is the major factor in the success of the total program. A therapist must be prepared to not only initially evaluate a patient but must also be adept at reevaluating the patient's condition at each stage. Body Techniques therapy does not provide a standard treatment protocol but rather presents a plan of application which allows the therapist to pick and choose the proper areas of treatment concentration and plan progression which will fit the individual patient. In other words, at no time should the therapist be locked into a treatment program which does not take into consideration the changing pattern of his patient's overall needs.

The case histories presented in this chapter illustrate the flexibility which is built into the program and stress the importance of the therapist's evaluative and judgmental capabilities.

Case History #1—Muscle Spasm/Triggerpoint

Patient G.E. arrived at our office with her mother and a friend. She had called earlier and her voice had revealed a deep concern as she described the pattern of pain in her neck and upper back. She indicated that she was a psychotherapist and was unable to fulfill her career responsibilities because of the excruciating pain. Since she had been unable to obtain relief through other means, she was advised to come into the office as soon as possible.

Initial Evaluation

Subjectively:
- Pain in the left upper back, between the shoulder blades, and around the cervical area
- Pain exacerbated by lifting and carrying books (a necessary activity as the patient was also teaching part-time at a local college)

Objectively:
- Palpation revealed muscle spasm in the left upper and right middle trapezius
- Muscle spasm at the medial border of the scapula
- Possible triggerpoint at the left scapula at the superior angle (There was an indication of a possible rather than a definite triggerpoint because it is usually impossible to positively identify a triggerpoint when a muscle is in spasm.)

Impression:
- The muscles of patient's left upper and right middle back were in spasm

Treatment

During the Initial Evaluation reassurance was given that the problem was due to muscle spasm and that at that time it was the only problem that could be detected. The diagnosis of muscle spasm was supported by the fact that G.E., being new at her career, was under intense pressure as she was experiencing some of the difficulties associated with administration and patient contact. One of her primary concerns was that her mother and friend would be apprised of the fact that such intense pain could be caused by muscle spasm. Apparently, since they had seen her as being unable to function in any role, they questioned that something as minor as a muscle spasm could be so debilitating.

The treatment rationale was explained, and it was also pointed out that head position and general posture were poor. If she wished to prevent any future recurrence of the muscle spasm it would be necessary to take her general posture into consideration. The therapeutic program consisted of two treatments.

Treatment #1: Cryotherapy to all muscles in spasm. (Ice pack was moved from the left cervical to the left mid-trapezius and rhomboid, to the left inferior muscles of the back, to the right mid-back.) These muscles were also electrically stimulated bilaterally. Body Techniques, prone and supine, with acupressure in the sitting positions, were applied. Instruction was given in the use of ice at home to be followed by the first two Body Movements (see page 81) and general range of motion exercises for loosening of the neck, shoulders, and scapula.

Patient G.E. followed through at home with ice and was experiencing "soreness" in the area but was pain-free when she returned for her second treatment.

Treatment #2: The patient received ice, pulsed Ultrasound to the triggerpoint that was present at the left superior angle of the scapula, electrical stimulation to the mid-back and cervical muscles, full Body Techniques, and correction in the Body Movements and range of motion exercises given in treatment number 1. The remainder of the Body Movements were taught. Her sitting posture was corrected because as a psychologist she was required to sit for extended periods. Instruction was also given in the techniques of correct general position during standing and walking and the proper method of carrying books. This postural information was reinforced through the Body Movements.

The patient was discharged and advised to contact the center if there was a recurrence of the spasm or pain.

Summary

Patient G.E. demonstrates a treatment protocol based on the Treatment of Pain Phase with the presenting symptomology being acute pain as a result of a functional problem. Consequently, treatment was given in the acute stage to *relieve the pain* from the muscle spasm (caused by tension and poor body alignment) and in the subacute stage to *reduce the spasm and triggerpoint* while educating the patient in all aspects of her particular postural problem areas. Since the pain had been eliminated and there was no major underlying dysfunction which required correction, Patient G.E. was dischargable after the second treatment. She had received a therapeutic exercise program aimed at reducing the tension level and postural strain, while simultaneously correcting general posture during functional activities.

Case History #2—Bilateral Lumbar Radiculitis

Patient C.A. was referred by a physician with the diagnosis of bilateral lumbar radiculitis. He was 28 years old, in excellent physical condition, and had been an athlete in college. Since that time he had continued on a physical fitness program which consisted of running (one-half hour a day, three times a week, without a good warm-up) and weight lifting on a personally owned machine which he used daily. The pain was not induced by acute trauma, and the patient was confused as to why it had occurred so suddenly. For the month prior to the initial appointment, normal functioning in any capacity had been impossible. Lying down produced the only pain relief whereas weight bearing caused an immediate exacerbation of the radiating pain and sitting was impossible. Therefore, this man was totally disabled with classical symptoms of a bilateral disc protrusion.

Initial Evaluation

Subjectively: The patient complained of intense low-back pain upon awakening which progressed to a painful condition that radiated to the buttocks and lower extremities bilaterally. Sitting, walking, or riding the bus to work caused an exacerbation of the disabling pain.

Objectively the following abnormalities were revealed:

- Triggerpoint in the left trapezius and occiput
- Muscle spasm in the right and left medial borders of the scapula
- Straight leg raise on the right leg = 73 degrees with pain in the low back
- Straight leg raise on the left leg = 78 degrees with pain in the low back
- Both hamstrings lacking in flexibility
- Crossover sign present on left SLR
- Rectus femoris: left, extreme lack of flexibility; right, within normal limits
- Muscle weakness: right hip abductor, left hip adductor, left hamstring. (Weakness was also indicated in the sit-up test for the abdominals but was misleading as this was not caused by a lack of strength in the abdominals but rather by the restricted range of movement in the low back which did not allow the patient the freedom of movement necessary to come to the sitting position.)
- Extreme lack of flexibility in: calves bilaterally and low back
- Inability of the lumbar curve to reverse
- Forward flexion limited to minus 10 inches from the floor
- Pelvis elevated 1 inch on the left side
- Lack of normal range of motion in the lumbar vertebrae

Impression

Patient C.A. was experiencing extreme lack of flexibility in the cervical, scapular, low back, bilateral calf, and left rectus femoris regions which was causing muscle spasm, triggerpoints, and radiating pain to the point of incapacitation.

Therapist's Thought Process

Biomechanically, this patient's key postural muscles are so lacking in flexibility that they are tilting and locking his pelvis in a forward tilt causing an increased lordosis and limiting joint movement in the lumbar area. The fact that the patient cannot actively reverse the curve is a major etiology of the radiating pain in the back and lower extremities. The tight and weak muscles that are listed in the Initial Evaluation are the cause of the pain superficially. However, the direct cause of the radiating pain is the fact that the increasing lordosis and immobile lumbar joints are putting pressure on adjacent nerve roots. In addition, the normal pelvic movement is further impeded by the general tightness of this patient. The initial goal of therapy therefore would be to decrease the pain by reducing the muscle spasm and triggerpoints. It will be necessary concurrently to begin to gently increase the flexibility of the low back, hamstrings, left rectus femoris, and the calf muscles. This secondary goal is crucial because, although this patient would receive relief of pain by merely treating the muscle spasm and triggerpoints, there would be an immediate return of the muscle spasm exacerbating the pain if his musculo-skeletal profile remained static. The therapist must continue to reduce the muscle spasm but at the same time must begin to loosen up the patient's low back so that proper placement of the pelvis can be encouraged. In this case, the Corrective Phase had to be initiated earlier to progress the patient more quickly through the Treatment of Pain Phase to a pain-free state. A program of therapy was begun and is outlined treatment by treatment in the following paragraphs.

Before Patient C.A.'s total program is illustrated, however, a mention must be made of the fact that on the day following the Initial Evaluation he called to relate that he had pulled a hamstring muscle. This produced an additional area of concentration which further complicated his musculo-skeletal profile. Therefore, it was necessary to spend some of the initial treatment time treating the pain and disability in the affected hamstring rather than concentrating on the areas designated in the Initial Evaluation.

Treatment Schedule

8/17—Patient received ice and electrical stimulation to his left hamstring at the site of the injury. He also received ice and pulsed Ultrasound for five minutes to a painful local spot on the low back. This was followed by the Medcolator to begin some work on the most apparent point of pain. (Patient could point to this spot on his left low back as being the most painful. There was so much pain during palpation that it was decided that Medcolator treatment alone would not break the triggerpoint; therefore, ice and pulsed Ultrasound were applied prior to the Medcolator.) Extensive instruction was given in the Head Wobble, Breathing, Neck Push, and Knees to Chest Body Movements in order to begin to break the spasm. A mild Hamstring Stretch was also added at this stage because in order to facilitate healing in the injured area the patient had to begin to bring the muscle to its resting length.

The Knees to Chest Body Movement was introduced at this time in order to bring the low-back muscles to their resting length to avoid spasm and to achieve one of the goals of the overall treatment by indirectly increasing flexibility in the low back. This patient was progressed more quickly through the treatment stages than normal because he had exercised extensively in the past, learned exercises quickly and well, and executed them correctly. The emphasis of his instruction was on breathing both independently as an exercise and as an adjunct to each exercise.

Patient C.A.'s first treatment also included prone and supine Body Techniques during the application of which two triggerpoints—one at the left occiput and the other in the left buttocks near the sacrum—were discovered. The patient was instructed to extensively ice the hamstring and the area of the left low back which was being worked on as well as any other area which produced pain. He was encouraged to do his exercises as often as possible with maximum emphasis on breathing and relaxation. (The Knees to Chest should be executed often in order to relieve pain as well as to keep the low-back muscles at their resting length.)

At the end of treatment number 1, Patient C.A. had received all that was necessary for pain control through the application of ice and the execution of Body Movements. Body Techniques were employed to help reduce the triggerpoints and muscle spasms that were present and to begin body awareness and postural training. They were also utilized as a main retrieval method for the therapist and provided further information of structural and soft tissue limitations. The information accumulated in this manner was used to develop the protocol for the next treatment.

8/19—Patient C.A. reported less-to-no pain in the low back area, a stiff neck, pain in the left cervical area, and pain in the hamstring. Since the previously discovered triggerpoint at the left occiput was still painful to palpation, it received Ultrasound. The Medcolator was applied to the low back and the buttocks. Ice was applied to the left cervical muscles and heat to the left hamstring (at different times). Heat was used on the hamstring because pain had diminished in that area and the goal at this point was to mildly stretch the muscle. An exercise review preceded the addition of the Neck Push, Pelvic Tilt, and Shoulder Wiggle (which the patient had difficulty doing). Instruction was given in two calf stretches—one to do at a desk and the other to be performed in the doorway with a towel. Body Techniques, prone and supine, and Bend-Sitting with the ethyl chloride spray were also included in this treatment session.

Mr. C.A. was followed through at home with cryotherapy; was executing all exercises and Body Movements correctly; and was working diligently on his prescribed stretches.

8/20—Patient continued to complain of hamstring pain and low-back tightness but not of low back or radiating pain. He received heat and Medcolator to the left hamstring and Medcolator to the low back followed by ice. Following a complete application of Body Techniques, the Plow was introduced.

Up to this time in Mr. C.A.'s therapeutic program, all of the movements and exercises had been indirectly affecting the area of concentration. Because the radiating pain had been eliminated, it was now safe to prescribe an exercise which would directly affect the area and progress the patient to the Corrective Phase of treatment. The Plow was being used to further stretch the low back muscles and encourage normal range of motion of the spinal joints because the patient was unable to perform the Bend-Sit exercise effectively due to the injured hamstring. (With an elderly or less active patient, however, this alternative exercise would be too strenuous.) At this stage in the treatment, tightness was still noticeable in the cervical and low back areas and the strong and tight cervical and shoulder muscles were locking the patient in extension at the OA joint and maintaining the head in the forward position.

8/23—Patient continued to present with three problem areas:
1. Triggerpoint, tightness, and lack of normal movement in the cervical area
2. Hamstring tear
3. Low back tightness with increased lordosis and right paraspinal spasm. (Work had been primarily done on the left side although the Medcolator had been applied to both. The right paraspinal muscle was rebelling against the stretching and therefore had to be treated.)

Patient subjectively reported that he felt great after Friday's treatment and had felt fine after stretching vigorously on Saturday. Upon awakening today (Monday) however, he had a recurrence of pain. When questioned he admitted that he had decreased the stretching on Sunday and his back had tightened up. This was a very effective teaching opportunity for the therapist to stress how important the follow-through stretching exercises were to the total program. The patient had been given an inkling into how well he could feel if he executed his program correctly and with regularity and had also discovered what would happen if he didn't carry out his responsibilities within the therapeutic program.

Ultrasound and heat were applied to the left hamstring because it was still bothersome. The low back and buttocks were treated with heat and Medcolator.

For the first time in Patient C.A.'s therapeutic program, heat was able to be applied due to the fact that he had been educated well enough at this stage to be able to control his own pain, to differentiate between pain and discomfort, and to discern whether the discomfort was due to muscle tightness rather than spasm or triggerpoint. Therefore, because the application of heat will add 15 percent elasticity to the muscle, it was the modality of choice to effect the treatment goal of stretching out the low-back muscles.

After heat and Medcolator were applied to the low back and buttocks, the patient received complete Body Techniques to balance soft tissue and skeletal body parts and to reinforce correct postural alignment. The home program was reviewed and, since he was going to be traveling on his honeymoon, the Standing Pelvic Tilt was added so that by holding this position when standing for long periods, C.A. could maintain the stretching gains previously made.

8/24—Patient reported increased pain upon awakening. It was explained that at this point his muscles were not stretched out to the extent that they would retain their new length constantly or for a long period of time. Therefore, when he felt them tightening up he had to intercede and stretch them out. During the night when there were few demands put upon his musculo-skeletal systems, his body would relax and his muscles would return to the shortened position to which they were accustomed.

This treatment session included cryotherapy, Ultrasound, Medcolator to the low-back spasm on the right side and to the left hamstring. (Working on the hamstring took valuable time away from treatment on the back but was necessary for patient relief.) Because the patient had difficulty doing the Standing Pelvic Tilt, after a review of all exercises, the therapist assisted him in executing the Plow. He was unable to assume the position of the exercise without assistance because his back was too tight and it caused pain similar to his original complaints.

8/25—Patient reported feeling great after stretching the night before. He experienced some stiffness but no pain in the low back upon arising. The fact that he was now awakening without pain was reassuring to the patient that substantial progress had been made. Treatment session included Medcolator to the left Hamstring; Ultrasound, ice, and Medcolator bilaterally to the mid-back; Medcolator to the buttocks; Body Techniques prone only; and a complete exercise review and explanation of the concept of the Standing Pelvic Tilt.

8/30—Patient reported feeling much better. Pain had decreased in the left hamstring as well as in the back in general. Palpation revealed tenderness and tightness in the right lower thoracic, lumbar, and buttocks areas. He received Medcolator to the buttocks and low back bilaterally, Ultrasound to the right lower thoracic and upper lumbar, prone and supine Body Techniques, Bend-sitting in the chair with ethyl chloride spray, and an exercise review. Patient C.A. had gained much more flexibility and was now performing the Standing Pelvic Tilt with ease. (The progress with this exercise was a dramatic functional example to the patient of his progress in general.)

The patient continued to make progress in his exercises, in how he was feeling, and in his ability to assume correct postural stances as he gained in flexibility. Posture was being taught throughout the treatment program in order to show the patient what to do with his body as he increased in his ability to move body parts previously limited.

8/31—The patient requested a more extensive program for his hamstring because he had no pain in the area and would be doing an increased amount of walking and standing on his honeymoon. Three additional Hamstring stretches were added as the injury had caused a decrease in pain-free flexibility to the muscle. There was no pain in the low back, unless the exercise routine was neglected for a day, although some stiffness remained upon awakening.

Medcolator with heat was applied to the hamstring because there was a concentration on that area during this treatment. This treatment session also included Medcolator to the low back; complete Body Techniques; and an exercise review. Patient C.A. was very confident that he could go on his honeymoon without concern because he had learned that his back pain was under his own control and as long as he continued to perform his exercises he would be pain-free and continue to progress in his condition in general. Should strain cause a recurrence of pain, C.A. was confident that his ice and exercise therapy would relieve him as it had done many times during the treatment program.

9/23—Patient C.A. returned after an absence of three and one-half weeks. He reported no low-back or hamstring pain while vacationing except while sitting on the plane. He had not exercised regularly since his last appointment but had done as much as possible. This treatment included Medcolator and heat to the low and mid-back, prone and supine Body Techniques, Bend-Sitting in the chair, a complete exercise review, and the addition of the Standing Side-Bend for lateral trunk flexibility. The Calf Stretches were progressed by placing a towel under the patient's feet to increase dorsi-flexion.

At this time, the patient had completed the Treatment of Pain Phase and presented with no major complaints but remained in the Corrective Phase because his underlying dysfunctions had not yet been resolved.

9/24—Patient received Medcolator with heat to the mid- and low back and full Body Techniques. During review of the Side Stretch, he was instructed to perform this exercise in front of a mirror in order to keep his weight from shifting or his rib cage from rotating while stretching. He continued to work diligently on all the previously prescribed stretches.

9/27—The patient complained of some discomfort in his mid-back. With palpation, a slight muscle spasm and triggerpoint on the left mid-thoracic area was detected.

This distress was not unusual because, when this much stretching is done and the low back lossens up, the stresses placed on the other areas of the back are changed and, consequently, these areas must readjust to new positions. Patient C.A.'s program was working by causing significant changes in his musculo-skeletal systems and he therefore had some tightening of the muscles in the mid-back area which caused discomfort and a triggerpoint.

Treatment included Ultrasound to the triggerpoint, ice and Medcolator to the area, full Body Techniques, and a complete exercise review. The therapeutic exercise program was progressed by the addition of the Springer's Stretch to stretch out the hip flexors and the quadriceps.

At this point in the Corrective Phase of treatment, Patient C.A. was progressing nicely. His program included Head Wobble, Breathing, Neck Push and Pelvic Tilt, Shoulder Wiggle, Knees to Chest, several Hamstring Stretches, two Calf Stretches, the Standing Side-Bend, the Plow, and the Sprinter's Stretch.

9/29—Patient still complained of discomfort in the thoracic area. Therefore, this treatment combined Ultrasound to the left upper thoracic and the thoracic paraspinals; Medcolator application to the mid- and low back; full Body Techniques; review of exercises; and correction of the Sprinter's Stretch and the Standing Side Bend. Several additional stretches for the hip flexor were given.

10/1—No complaints were presented other than a mild discomfort in the left upper thoracic paraspinal. Patient received Ultrasound to this area; Medcolator to the mid- and low back; heat to the low back; and full Body Techniques. A Scapula Pull was added since there was a problem in the upper back. A total exercise review was done which included a correction of the Plow which would enable stretching of the upper and lower back. The Roman Chair routine (see page 102) was introduced and these same exercises were performed at home crosswise on a bed with someone stabilizing his feet. The discomfort in the thoracic area was due to his incorrect posture during daily activities and also because of the long-standing tightness on this area caused by the extensive weight lifting he had done.

10/4—Medcolator and ice was applied to the mid-thoracic area along with Body Techniques, prone and supine, and another complete exercise review. Posture review and control was also stressed at this time. It was noted that the left hip flexor had been loosened sufficiently by the action of the previously prescribed stretches. In addition, the patient received an extension exercise done over the arm of a sofa or back of a straight chair which would mobilize the mid-thoracic area because the muscular exercise program had not *completely* eradicated the discomfort in this area.

Patients who are involved in such an extensive stretching program of maintenance to do at home are benefited greatly if the therapist includes extra exercises which can be done during the daily routine. Therefore, Patient C.A. was given his traditional home exercise program but for his trouble areas he was also taught several exercises which could be done at a desk, in a chair, in the elevator, against the wall, etc. Effective therapy can only be achieved by including many different avenues of approach for working on a patient's areas of concentration. The therapeutic exercise program must be flexible in order to meet the needs of busy people who can often regress in their recovery by missing a day's home follow-through due to lack of time. A few alternative exercises can fill the gap if it is absolutely necessary to miss the full regimen.

At this time, Patient C.A. brought in literature concerning the weight system that he had been using at home. A program was devised which would allow him to work independently on this weight machine to strengthen the areas of muscle weakness which had been discovered during the Initial Evaluation. This type of strengthening was appropriate at this time because the patient was free of pain and was doing extensive stretching on the Roman Chair. It was time to introduce the strengthening exercises which would affect the weak muscles discovered during the Initial Evaluation and in so doing the patient would be progressed to the Preventive Phase of his individualized treatment program. In retesting for forward flexion at this time, Patient C.A. was able to touch his fingertips to the floor whereas initially he was minus 10 inches in forward flexion. This retesting afforded the patient a vivid illustration of the degree of functional improvement which had been acquired through his own efforts and an effective physical therapy program.

10/6—The patient had virtually no pain; was doing very well; his posture had improved; he was happy; and he requested and was given a posture pillow to be used at work until he could strengthen the thoracic area. He received Medcolator with heat, Body Techniques, and a complete review of exercises.

10/7—Patient received Medcolator on the low back and buttocks; heat; Body Techniques; and a complete review of exercises. He was instructed that his future program should include his therapeutic exercise program; a weight lifting program for the three weak muscles; incorporation of the proper posture into his daily living; and a gradual return to all other normal activities. The patient was discharged at this time, pain-free and armed with all pertinent information for his preventive maintenance program.

The restorative stage of the Corrective Phase began when the strengthening exercises were prescribed for Patient C.A., and he began to return gradually to his weight program. He progressed into the Preventive Phase when he began to engage in some of the activities that he had done previous to the initial bout of low-back pain and dysfunction. Initially, the re-introduction of these activities should only be allowed under the guidance of the therapist as modifications are usually required to avoid strain and pain recurrence. When people perform general exercises like jogging, racewalking, swimming, or running, they usually use incorrect technique and improper posture which places biomechanical stress on certain body parts. Either they begin a vigorous program of exercise with existing mechanical imbalances, do not stretch out properly, warm up or cool down correctly, or execute the stroke or lift incorrectly. It is the therapist's job to advise the patient in the correct execution of these activities in order to prevent future strain.

The phases of treatment are not clear-cut. Even though the patient progresses through the phases, there is not a clear-cut delineation as to when one ends and the next begins, as one phase usually carries over into the next. The Treatment of Pain Phase is carried throughout the therapeutic program regardless of what phase of correction or prevention the patient has attained. It is understandable then, why handing a patient an exercise program to perform on his own doesn't work and is an ineffective method of health care. If Patient C.A. had been given the entire set of exercises in one or two sessions and then sent on his way, his condition would have become much worse. This is true because even though he would have had the exact same set of exercises, he would have been denied the knowledge, skill, and guidance of the therapist in treating the conditions that arose because of the exercise program itself. As the body parts are readjusted to achieve proper alignment and biomechanical forces shift, the soft tissue and skeletal systems are forced to accommodate new and different stresses and therefore the therapist must be available to evaluate and treat these changes. The odds are completely against a patient who receives a limited, nonindividualized, undirected program of treatment. Not only will he not recover, but he will be convinced that physical therapy has nothing to offer him.

Summary

This young man exhibited symptoms of a condition which often receives surgical intervention. The severe radiating pain which was exacerbated by weight bearing and relieved by lying down is typical symptomology of a bilateral disc protrusion. However, after 16 treatments of the Body Techniques program, the patient was asymptomatic and had returned to all functional and recreational activity.

Case History #3—Long-Standing and Recurrent Back Pain

Patient K.J. is 40 years old and a perfect specimen of a well-conditioned, middle-aged man. He is a teacher of the martial arts and exercises three hours a day. His back problem had been a constant companion for the last 20 years, having its initial introduction during his Marine Corps service. An extensive variety of treatments had been prescribed and undergone over the years with the most recent being three years of chiropractic. In the past year, K.J. had been plagued with a series of job-related injuries and had been receiving workmen's compensation for several months. At the time of the Initial Evaluation, he was back at work but still in pain and under the care of a chiropractor. His main concerns were his inability to function normally and the restrictions his back limitations placed upon his athletic performance.

Initial Evaluation

Patient has experienced life-long back pain and has had treatment by numerous doctors and chiropractors with the realization of only short term relief. The last traumatic incident was approximately one month ago. The following abnormalities were found in his musculo-skeletal evaluation:

- Subjective report of pain in the small of his back, especially on the left side with radiation to his left buttock and down to his left knee

- Triggerpoint at the medial border of the right scapula
- Muscle spasm in the left low-back paravertebral muscle
- Three inches from the floor in forward flexion
- Normal pelvic rhythm was absent during the forward flexion test
- Hamstring flexibility: right = 65 degrees; left = 73 degrees. (The hamstring test on the left evoked pain across the patient's low back.)
- Positive straight leg raise on the left
- Forward head position with a triggerpoint at the right occiput
- OA joint lacking in range of motion because of extremely tight and strong cervical muscles which were pulling patient into the forward head position and locking him there
- Limited internal and external rotation of both hips
- Left rectus femoris was extremely limited in flexibility
- Severe bilateral range of motion limitation in hip joints
- Muscle weakness in: left adductor; right abductor; left hamstring; low back
- Standing side bend indicated left side tightness
- Left calf muscle was extremely tight

Initial Problem Areas for Consideration:

- Right and left hips which are extremely limited in flexibility (concentration on the left)
- Left side of the trunk which is severely limited in flexibility
- Low back which is tight with weakness in the intrinsic muscles of the lumbar curve
- Right scapula because of the triggerpoints and the muscle spasms present
- Cervical muscles because they are very tight and overdeveloped. The limited range of motion of the joints—especially the OA joint—is locking this patient in the forward head position. This is also reinforcing his tight low back because the forward head position causes increased strain and lack of normal movement in the lumbar area.

Treatment Goals:

The *initial goal* for this patient was to decrease his pain and reduce whatever triggerpoints and muscle spasms were present. The *secondary goal* was to assist the patient in achieving normal flexibility in the areas of concentration listed in the Initial Evaluation. The *ultimate goal* was to increase the strength in the weakened areas and correct the overall body positioning so that a pain-free, normal level of functioning could be obtained.

Treatment Plan

Patient K.J.'s initial program consisted of cryotherapy, electrotherapy, Body Techniques, postural alignment, and Body Movements to help decrease the pain along with the early introduction of Ultrasound to reduce the triggerpoints. Due to the fact that this patient had achieved only short-lived relief from pain in the past, it was felt that something should be done early in the program to show him that the therapy could do more than just temporarily blot out his symptoms. Therefore, for motivational considerations, it was necessary to illustrate the corrective aspects of the program much earlier in this patient's treatment plan than is normally the case.

In checking the Initial Evaluation it was noted that the pelvis was tilted in a manner which increased the lumbar lordosis and the forward head position exacerbated the problem. Also the strength and tightness of the low-back muscles reinforced this position and put pressure on the nerve or nerve root which was causing both the recurring muscle spasm in the back and the radiating pain. Because it was advantageous to the patient to do something quickly to reverse this condition and to illustrate that something was being done to correct the underlying problem, the Sprinter's Stretch was given which would begin to loosen up both hips.

After the first week of treatments, patient K.J. was complaining that he could see no benefit from the treatment program. Upon investigation a surprising fact was revealed. The patient admitted that he had not followed through at home with the exercise program prescribed. Upon further questioning it was deduced that, because of the long-term nature of the problem and the previous treatments of passive mode which he had been subjected to, Patient K.J. had not grasped the essential nature of his active role in his own treatment. After the therapist reiterated the need for home reinforcement of the therapeutic gains made in the treatment room and the essential nature of patient participation in the program, the advances in Patient K.J.'s condition were rapid and obvious. He received 24 treatments to correct a wide range of problems and the swiftness of the success (discharged in three months) was due to the efforts of this patient. His hard work—exercising three hours a day in the prescribed manner—enabled him to achieve his ultimate goal in a remarkably short time.

The second week of treatment concentrated on the tightness in the left hip flexor and quadricep because that was an important contributing factor to the pain in the left low back. Treatment consisted of:

Ultrasound to the left low back where a palpable spot had been isolated along the lumbar vertebrae at the attachment of the hip flexor; Medcolator to the low back; Medcolator to the left hip flexor and quadricep as high as possible to the hip joint; and Body Techniques, prone and supine.

Because this patient was accustomed to an extensive exercise program, a greater amount of home exercise was prescribed in a shorter time than was normal for the non-athletic patient. Patient K.J.'s program consisted of cryotherapy followed by the Head Roll, the Neck Push, Breathing and Relaxation, the Hip Flexor Stretch on the edge of the bed, the Sprinter's Stretch, and two Calf Stretches.

Each progressive treatment session found a patient subjectively reporting physical strides and emotional contentment with the program. Transitory muscle spasms were treated and the home exercise program was expanded to include the Hip Roll, Hip Extension on three pillows, and an Adductor Stretch (see Figures 1 and 2) to improve rotation of the hips. In this exercise, the patient squats down with the soles of his feet on the floor, heels touching and toes pointing outward. His elbows are placed close to the knees on the inside of his thighs. The patient merely leans his weight forward which encourages external rotation and stretches both the adductors and internal rotators of the hips. This exercise was added to Mr. K.J.'s program because limitation around the hip areas was a major etiology of his back problem. Concurrently, the Knees to Chest and the Plow were added to his program to stretch out the low back.

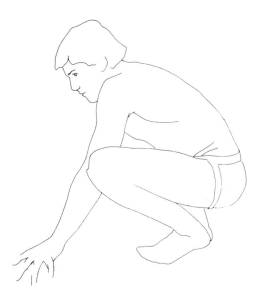

Figure 1

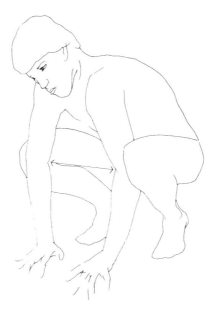

Figure 2

The Plow is executed by lying on your back and bringing your legs overhead while keeping them straight and touching your knees to the mat. Initially this exercise frightened the patient because he felt a strain in his problem area. However, with proper guidance in the use of deep breathing and relaxation, he was taught to "work through" the restrictive tissue. K.J. gradually gained more confidence in the exercise as the therapist illustrated different ways to stretch the various areas of the spine in order to make this exercise specific to stretching out the low back. Patient K.J.'s problem was being worked on from two different approaches, both superior and inferior to the pelvis. Therefore the areas were being balanced that were restricting normal movement of the pelvis where the major muscles attach at the low back and around the legs and hips.

During one of the treatment evaluations it was noticed that the patient was overstretching and therefore was creating undue soreness in his back. This was remedied by slowing the patient down in his execution of the stretching exercises, by working on coordinating his breathing more fully, and by making sure that he wasn't bouncing or forcing the stretch. He was taught to work into and breathe through the stretch in a coordinated manner in order to do these exercises correctly. Progressing well in his program, as he began to stretch out the low back, a triggerpoint was discovered directly above the right iliac crest. This was reduced by the application of Ultrasound followed by Medcolator, heat, and an application of Body Techniques. The modalities had been changed from ice to heat because the patient was bothered merely by soreness and not by pain and the heat would be a positive force in reducing the soreness and stretching the muscle.

Psychologically, Patient K.J. was still not completely convinced that the program of treatment was the answer for him even though he was conscious of the changes being realized in his body by the treatment protocol. Although the pain was decreased, he was constantly expecting it to return because for the last 20 years the standard route had been that the pain would begin to disappear and then would reappear. It was the therapist's job at each session to give the degree of explanation, reinforcement, and moral support necessary to assure the patient that this particular therapy was going to work for him and that it would be this individualized approach which would produce total recovery. He needed to be educated in the fact that the stretching exercises would produce soreness in the muscles being stretched and that this was a sign of progression not regression. He also had to be made aware of the fact that initially his muscles could be expected to go into a fatigued state after normal use because these muscles were not accustomed to operating throughout the entire range of motion. When these newly stretched muscles were reeducated and strengthened by the conditioning program to be prescribed, the patient would be able to put larger demands upon them without soreness or pain. Up until that time, however, he was vulnerable to strain and muscle spasm from overuse or misuse. Although this patient originally seemed to be prepared for the demands of the therapeutic program, it soon became obvious that the years of non-successful treatments and recurring frustration had produced a patient physically able to execute the therapeutic program but psychologically unable to expect full recovery. K.J. was also more sensitive to the discomforts which accompany the corrective exercises and misread them as a negative rather than a positive sign. The psychological demands of the Body Techniques program were heavily felt by the therapist during the treatment of this particular patient because of the added support he needed to progress through the Corrective Phase.

During treatment number 12, Patient K.J. asked for permission to run. Since there had been no complaint of pain for the last three or four days and the therapeutic exercise program was progressing nicely, permission was given for a once-a-day run of under two miles, accompanied by complete stretching before and after the run. (Patient had been accustomed to running for five to ten miles a day.)

Treatment number 10 saw the introduction of the Roman Chair routines during which the patient stretched out both sides of his trunk with primary work being done on the left where there was an area of increased tightness. During session number 12, he requested an exercise to strengthen the abdominals. In attempting to introduce the Sit Up/Sit Back abdominal strengthening exercise, it became evident that the patient was unable to assume the position of a normal lumbar curve because he was unable to arch his back in the sitting position. Once the muscles were stretched out in that area it was obvious that he had very little movement in the lumbar segments. Since it was necessary to increase the range of motion of the lumbar vertebrae, Patient K.J. was given a routine of extension exercises. The treatment sessions also included Ultrasound to the triggerpoint at the right iliac crest and a hot pack and electrotherapy to the low back. Exercises continued to be added quickly and, at treatment number 14 a stretch was introduced which would increase the range of motion of the shoulders and stretch out the pectoral muscles. Because this patient had been in the forward head position and had maintained an immobile lumbar curve for such an extended period of time, his shoulders had become somewhat protracted. This condition was reinforced by ultrastrong pectoral muscles which had been strengthened through previous weight training. However, the limitation was muscular only and normal shoulder range of motion was gained in less than one week of vigorous stretching.

On treatment 15, the patient requested permission to resume weight training. This was granted for the arms and chest but was not yet permitted for the lower extremities. Because the therapeutic program was concentrating on stretching out the hip flexors, the quadriceps, and the hamstrings, these areas were not ready to be strengthened at this time. Heavy weight training in these areas would be counter-productive and would negate the strides made with previous stretching.

At treatment session 16, Patient K.J. was feeling extremely well. He was able to run, stretch, and use free weights for his upper body without causing low-back pain. Complaints of occasional soreness, which both patient and therapist attributed to the massive stretching program, were easily alleviated by modality applications. At this time, an Adductor Stretch with Pelvic Rotation in Standing Position was added to the program (see Figures 3 and 4). The Neck Push was being worked on rigorously to assist the patient in reversing the forward head position and was frequently producing a stiff neck which was relieved by the Medcolator and a hot pack. Another Hip Flexor Stretch using a chair was introduced and was executed by placing one foot on a chair and extending the other foot. The stretch was then accomplished by dropping the body weight at a triangular point between the rear foot and the chair.

Previous to treatment number 18, Patient K.J. went sky diving

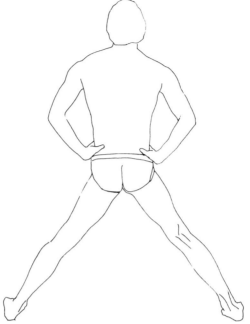

Figure 3

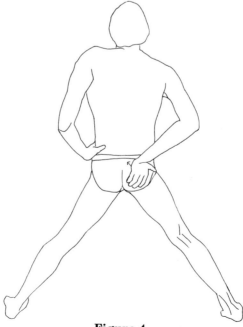

Figure 4

(contrary to recommendation), and this caused him to complain of pain in the lower chest which was attributed to the fact that he had hit the ground with too much force. This pain precluded stretching activity for a few days; therefore, his home exercise program was discontinued until the 20th visit.

During the reevaluation period of the 20th treatment session, the therapist motivated the patient by telling him that he could be discharged from treatment when he could return to his regular regimen of judo practice without experiencing low-back pain. It was disclosed that the judo practice had been secretly attempted a week earlier and at that time pain had been experienced. Upon further questioning, it became apparent to both parties that the patient had experienced merely soreness in the low back and not pain. However, because of the previous 20 years of pain, it was difficult for Patient K.J. to differentiate between the two conditions. He also could not understand his continued inability to perform judo movements when he was able to execute such a wide range of exercises. This inconsistency was explained when, while attempting once again to place the patient in the position for the Sit Up/Sit Back exercise, it became apparent that the patient currently had the necessary range of motion, but the intrinsic muscles of the lumbar area were not strong enough to hold the lumbar curve. These muscles had not contracted fully for a long period of time because of the limited range of motion available in the lumbar vertebrae and the static position of the patient's pelvis. The patient was beginning to make gains in this area however, because he had worked diligently until he could hold the lumbar curve in the preliminary sit back position. This indicated a major breakthrough in Patient K.J.'s therapy. Since it was agreed upon that increased strength in the intrinsic muscles would allow the patient to engage in all of his activities without the soreness (that he still called "pain") in his low back, the major thrust of therapy and the home program would be continuation of the stretching with heavy emphasis on the Sit Up/Sit Back exercise.

During the 23rd treatment, Patient K.J. complained that he had attempted to practice judo and again had to stop because of increased pain in his back. The therapist requested a demonstration of the pain-producing judo moves and the patient was able to duplicate these without an exacerbation of pain. This discrepancy in pain appearance was attributed to two factors. During a judo workout the intrinsic low-back muscles become fatigued and are overworked before the moves illustrated by the patient are even attempted. In contrast, when the patient performs in the therapist's office, his muscles are warm, relaxed, and rested and therefore are able to tolerate the demands made upon them. Second, Patient K.J. had developed a conditioned response which had been created by 20 years of pain. Several times during the therapeutic program he had commented that he had had the pain for a long time and that he could not just get it out of his head. The pain had become so much a part of his life that it was expected under certain circumstances. He indicated that it would take time for his mind to realize what his back already knew and that was that the pain was truly gone and, if the program of maintenance was continued regularly, would remain a memory rather than a reality.

Even though the patient was pain-free, motivated, and educated enough to be discharged at this time, the therapist extended the therapy by three sessions in order to psychologically prepare the patient for discharge. These treatments included an extensive exercise review and a strong reinforcement of the fact that Mr. K.J. was no longer a patient with a medical "back problem" but rather a healthy individual who was receiving a highly individualized conditioning program for an active life. Encouragement was given to reduce the strains of the previous levels of judo performance by easing back on the intensity of participation since this appeared to be the only activity in which soreness occurred. Eventually this soreness would be alleviated by the strengthening of the intrinsic muscles of the low back and full participation would become possible.

Patient K.J. was discharged in excellent physical condition after 24 treatments. He had progressed from a discouraged, pain-plagued, workmen's compensation case to a pain-free, active man who had normal flexibility and muscle strength in every muscle in which he had been limited except the intrinsic of the lumbar curve. This corrected musculo-skeletal profile allowed the patient an intact body posture for all activities. He was now able to run five to seven miles a day, lift weights, box, execute a one-to-two hour stretching program, work, and in general live a restriction-free life. The only remaining area of weakness, the intrinsic muscles, would be treated by the Sit Up/Sit Back exercise in conjunction with a continuation of the exercise routine utilizing the free weights and Universal equipment which he had at his disposal.

Summary

Patient K.J. is an example of a chronic problem which created numerous musculo-skeletal abnormalities over a long period of time even though the patient was generally well-conditioned and healthy. The treatment of this patient combined the physical skills and psychological facets of the Body Techniques program. Heavy emphasis was placed upon the individualized psychological approach which the therapist must continually keep in mind while preparing the therapeutic treatment program for each patient. The rapid advances gained in this particular patient's condition were made possible by his thoroughly cooperative and active participation and desire to think health rather than sickness.

Because he was a patient who wished to control his own body, it was expedient for the therapist to help him overcome 20 years of the mental conditioning that he had a "back problem." The therapy would have been neither as effective nor as rapid if Patient K.J.'s psychological needs had been overlooked.

Case History #4—Scoliosis and Hypertrophied Transverse Process L5

Ms. K.L. was referred with a diagnosis of lumbar radiculitis. She is in her 30s, a movie producer, and prior to her back injury had led an active life which included swimming, yoga (at least five times a week) and total absorption in a highly stressful career. Two immediately obvious components of this patient's psychological profile were her strongly emotional personality and the self-imposed pressure caused by an intense desire for career and material success. She had a history of mild and vague low-back discomfort which flared into total incapacitating pain during a yoga session when her back went into spasm. At that time an orthopedist prescribed bed rest, analgesics, and eventually resumption of mild activity with a corset. This therapy did not prove to be effective and consequently a doctor of physical therapy at one of New York's leading hospitals was consulted. While under his care, Ms. K.L. received physical therapy for three months. At the end of this period, the excruciating pain originally experienced had been alleviated; however, the patient felt that the three-month investment in rehabilitation had not produced an acceptable level of functional recovery. On the recommendation of a friend, Ms. K.L. requested a referral of her case for our consideration.

Initial Evaluation

Patient K.L. presented with a six-month-old back problem. The impression that she was doomed to be a cripple for the rest of her life had produced severe psychological distress. Although the problem had been diagnosed as serious, there had been no enlightenment as to the etiology of the symptoms other than the possibility of a herniated disk which was causing the lumbar radiculitis. The Initial Evaluation revealed the following musculo-skeletal profile:

- Subjective report of pain in the left low back radiating to the left buttock and continuing to the left knee. This pain was intense enough to completely restrict activity.
- X-rays showed a hypertrophied transverse process at L5, left side
- Atrophy of the right paraspinal muscle
- Pelvic rotation to the right with elevation on the left

- Leg length discrepancy: right leg ¾ inch longer than left
- Left buttock was weak and mush
- General asymmetry of posture
- Extreme tightness of the left side of the back

Palpation was the primary vehicle for discovering the abnormalities in the soft tissue as well as the skeletal system. The right paraspinal muscle had atrophied and the left paraspinal muscle was of a hard consistency (not in spasm, just in a gristly state). Most of the pain was experienced on the left side of the trunk, lateral to the spinal column, where consistency of the muscles was very different from the right side. Therefore, this patient presented with the following concurrent abnormalities:

- Congenital and functional skeletal problems
- Soft tissue dysfunction of muscles not working effectively for such a long period of time that their consistency had changed and had become very painful
- A serious postural position that was exacerbating the symptoms
- Overall limitation in function

Ms. K.L. was caught in a vicious cycle in which the less activity she engaged in to prevent aggravation of the condition, the more severe the symptomology.

Treatment Plan

The initial plan of treatment was to decrease the pain; however, the protocol would differ in this patient because the problem was not merely caused by a muscle spasm but rather by muscle spasm superimposed upon other soft tissue abnormalities. It was decided that, since in the previous therapy program Patient K.L. had received electrotherapy for three months and had experienced only a moderate amount of relief, Ultrasound treatments would be the first modality used in the Treatment of Pain Phase. Therefore, pulsed Ultrasound was applied to the left low back followed by ice packs and Medcolator on the right and left sides. During this first treatment, a triggerpoint was discovered at the left low back around the iliac crest which Ultrasound reduced. After an application of prone and supine Body Techniques, the patient was introduced to the Head Wobble, Breathing and Relaxation, Neck Push, Pelvic Tilt, Combination, and Hip Extension on two pillows. This patient had exercised extensively in the past so she could be introduced to these Body Movements quickly.

Treatment session number 2 found the patient reporting some pain relief and an enjoyment derived from doing the Body Movements in a new and concentrated manner. She indicated that even though the Body

Movements did not entirely differ from the exercises she had been previously exposed to, the manner of execution was definitely unique and therefore beneficial. This difference was manifested in two areas: 1) the use of breathing and relaxation methods of movement; and 2) the two-stage aspect of each exercise, i.e., the position the patient assumes and the energy that the patient directs to a specific area of concentration to accomplish a change in the body condition. This treatment session also included Ultrasound to the triggerpoint and the left side, ice and Medcolator to the low back and buttocks, prone and supine Body Techniques, Bend-Sit with spray (page 44), and instruction in the Cat Back exercise.

During the 3rd treatment session, Patient K.L. indicated that she felt that she was receiving benefit from the treatment and that the therapy was not only different but specific and directed to the point of her areas of concentration. However, this sense of well-being had caused her to put in an extremely long and stressful day at work which resulted in an exacerbation of pain. Therefore, pulsed Ultrasound was applied to the lumbar area and the left iliac crest. Ice, prone and supine Body Techniques, Bend/Sit, and an introduction to the Standing Pelvic Tilt comprised the therapeutic program for this treatment.

At this time it was suggested that the patient take some time off from work to rest and concentrate on her therapy. However, due to contract negotiations, she was unable to do so at this particular time. The therapist reminded her that the physical and emotional demands placed on her by her career were working in direct contrast to the principles of the treatment program and therefore, she was not receiving full benefit from the therapy.

Treatment sessions 4 and 5 consisted of pulsed Ultrasound to the left low back and the left iliac crest, Medcolator and ice to the low back and cervical muscles, and full Body Techniques with a concentration on the lumbar area. Side lifts with two pillows under the knees were added to the home program.

On the 6th treatment the patient's symptoms had subsided substantially but she still continued to complain of a very deep ache or pain in the left low back. In a reassessment of the treatment protocol, the therapist decided to continue Ultrasound because of the pain relief it afforded the patient. It was also discovered that the hip flexor was much more involved than originally thought and that the quadratus lumborum on the left side needed more intense treatment. Therefore, Patient K.L. received deep acupressure along the lumbar vertebrae in hopes that this would reach critical parts of those muscles. Pulsed Ultrasound was applied to as much of the muscle as possible. Fibrositis and connective tissue massage was given in the area of the left low back. Two exercises were added to reinforce the goals of this session, i.e., the Knee Drop (see Figures 5, 6, and 7) and the Standing Side-Bend. The introduction of the Standing Side-Bend (see Figures 8 and 9) to both sides illustrated a noticeable difference between the two. When the patient bent over to the right side, she had an intense pulling on the left because the muscles were abnormal. When she bent over to the left side, she experienced excruciating pain which was attributed to her hypertrophic transverse process and the inflamed area around it. Therefore, she was instructed to do this exercise in a very controlled manner by executing it only to the point of pain and then stopping. Eventually, after several months, both sides were without pain.

Because Patient K.L. continued to present a localized pain in the area of the hypertrophic transverse process, it was decided that her inflammation might be decreased by a cortisone injection and steps were taken to arrange an appointment with her personal physician. The patient voiced reservations concerning this recommendation, however, since all parties

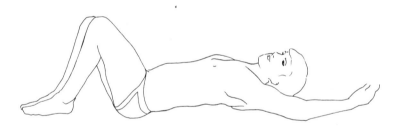

Figure 5

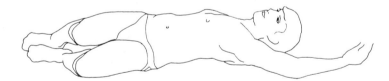

Figure 6

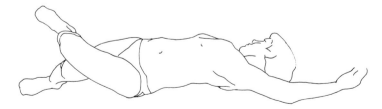

Figure 7

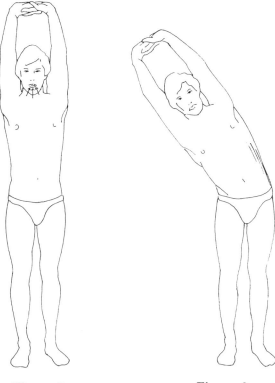

Figure 8   **Figure 9**

(the patient, therapist, and physician) agreed that this area appeared to be holding up progress in the program, it seemed wise to resort to an injection of an anti-inflammatory agent. This 9th session also included the addition of specific mobilization to the left hip because it was lacking in range of motion.

The cortisone was injected by the patient's physician two treatments later and produced a negative response which caused total physical and mental incapacitation. Therefore, after a two-day hiatus, the injected area was again treated with Ultrasound. The patient received Medcolator to the low back and buttocks, acupressure to the area, prone and supine Body Techniques, and Bend-Sitting in a chair. *All patients receive Body Techniques throughout their entire program of treatment to help normalize the skeletal system and soft tissue and to work toward an improved body placement.*

During treatment number 15, while applying Body Techniques, the therapist noticed that as the patient's left scapula was mobilized the identical pain in the left low back reappeared. The observation was made

that the latissimus dorsi muscle was adhesed from the inferior angle of
the scapula through the lumbar area to the iliac crest. To help relieve this
restriction, the Roman Chair was introduced and the patient was
instructed in the side stretches in order to get a deeper stretch on the left
side. This stretching was done with extreme care, with careful attention
to patient positioning, and with an application of ethyl chloride to
prevent further spasm of irritable musculature and an exacerbation of
pain.

Patient K.L. began treatment on November 30 with severe problems in
multi-affected areas. On February 1, she was ecstatic about her progress
and the therapist continued the modality and therapeutic exercise
program treating spasms and triggerpoints as they arose. A severe
emotional stress exacerbated the pain on February 19, but this was able
to be reduced quickly with Body Techniques, relaxation therapy, and
modality applications. The patient's progress was continually being
hampered by the demands she insisted on placing upon her body through
the hectic schedule she kept both at work and in her personal life.

On March 1, a recheck of the patient's progress and present condition
was made. It is important to point out that since the superficial problems
had, at this point, been successfully eliminated, the therapist was able to
discern additional areas of concentration need. This reevaluation discovered weakness in the left hip abductor and increased tightness in the left
rectus femoris. The tightness was treated by the addition of a prone
Rectus Femoris Stretch (see Figure 10) with one pillow under the knee of
the side being stretched. During the execution of this exercise, the
patient's left low back area went into spasm. This provided further
substantiation of the diagnosis that the hip flexor was one of the sources
of the major underlying problem causing the superficial symptomology.
Ms. K.L. was given the Hip Flexor Exercise on the left in a position which

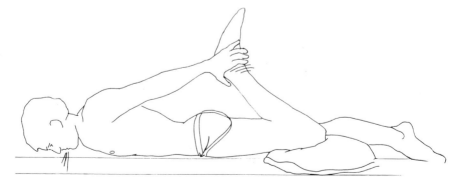

Figure 10

caused as little pain as possible. She was also taught how to ease into and control the stretch by using correct breathing techniques. This is an example of how a corrective exercise, even though it causes pain, must be and can be safely executed if a patient is instructed properly.

The next treatment progression was initiated on March 8 through the addition of a progressive resistance exercise of the hip abductor on the left leg with a five pound weight with rapid repetitions followed by isometrics at the end of the range. Additional weight was added on successive days during the supervised treatment time.

At this time, career responsibilities required Patient K.L. to fly to California. She returned with glowing reports of a full week of pain-free, normal activity. However, on the day that she had returned, the patient had turned in an extension-rotation type movement and her hip flexor had gone into spasm. The Ultrasound and Medcolator were ineffective in releasing the spasm and eradicating the pain; however, relief was obtained by having the patient side-lie on the right while holding her left leg in abduction and extension. This position not only relieved the pain in the leg and the buttock but also stretched the hip flexor. The spasm reconfirmed that the hip flexor was a major source of the patient's problem. Slightly stretching this area and bringing it back to its resting length by utilizing the breathing techniques, while at the same time protecting the back and lumbar areas, gave this patient relief from the pain. Patient K.L. was constantly being educated in the proper methods of pain relief in the event that she might need to employ them at home or while traveling and was a willing participant in her home exercise follow-up routine.

Because the left low back area was still a source of discomfort, even though it was not an area of severe restriction, an examination of this area was necessary to ascertain what was prohibiting complete recovery. The therapist accomplished this examination by placing Patient K.L. in a right, side-lying position with her left leg stretched over a pillow. While in this position, through palpation, very deep muscle spasms and a trigger-point were discovered along the left bottom rib posteriorly. It was also found that the intrinsic muscles in the back were in spasm. The only way these deep muscle areas could be felt was to position the patient correctly or to stretch her out on the Roman Chair to eliminate the tightness from the superficial muscles.

On March 26, the patient reported that she had been in increased pain in the last three days. This was in conjunction with a generalized feeling of wooziness which seemed to foretell the onset of a viral infection. Because an increase in back pain is often the case when a patient experiences a general malaise, the symptoms did not indicate treatment change except for a lighter application of Body Techniques and no strenuous exercise. The standard treatment relieved the pain symptomatology.

On March 29, Patient K.L. reported an exacerbation of pain since the last treatment which constant ice packs had not reduced. This was an unusual turn in the progressive flow and demanded intense evaluation. Upon questioning, the patient admitted that she had carried something heavy and immediately her back had gone into spasm. Patients are particularly vulnerable when they begin to feel better because as they approach a state of normality they usually overdo and cause a temporary physical setback with the accompanying mental frustration. Ms. K.L.'s overload had caused recurrence of the low-back pain with numbness and radiation to the left leg. Upon inspection and palpation, the quadratus lumborum was found to be in spasm and three triggerpoints were evident. Pulsed Ultrasound was applied to the left paraspinal and along the left iliac crest followed by Body Techniques. The Sprinter's Hip Flexor Stretch (see Figures 11 and 12) was added to the program because the patient's left side exhibited a great degree of tightness.

The effective therapist keeps a patient apprised at all times of the reasoning behind the prescribed program. In Patient K.L.'s particular case, she was constantly being reminded that the exercises were chosen for her because she needed to stretch her left hip flexor; because her low back must be equalized through the side stretching; and because each

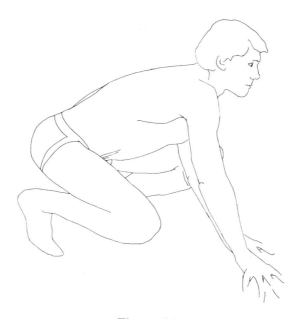

Figure 11

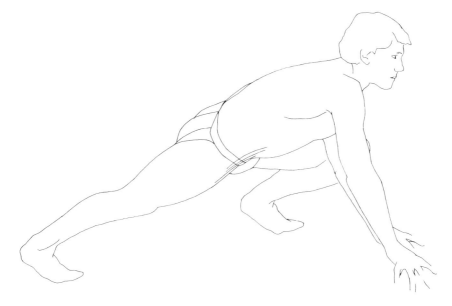

Figure 12

exercise had a goal that fit in with the total picture and the individual treatment goal needed at the particular stage of progress she had attained.

On April 5, which was less than a week after she had been given the Sprinter's Hip Flexor Stretch, the patient was very much improved. The rest that she had taken plus the stretch had alleviated, by her own estimation, about 75% of the pain. The therapist applied the same modalities with a change to heat instead of ice as the pain was relieved and stretching was the primary goal. Body Techniques were followed by another Hip Flexor Stretch at the edge of the bed which was merely another of the several ways that the area of concentration was being affected. The patient agreed to take a week's rest during which time she was to work actively on her total program.

On April 16, Patient K.L. returned showing great improvement in her condition. Palpation revealed no tightness, spasm, or tenderness to touch for the first time. The main complaint was in the left hip abductor and the left abdominal oblique muscle. Treatment consisted of pulsed Ultrasound to the left low back and superior iliac crest; heat and Medcolator to the left buttock and left abductor; and mobilization of the left hip. The only daily activities which caused any back discomfort were those involved with sitting and carrying. Therefore, the therapist analyzed the patient's sitting position and corrected it, restricting the length of time for sitting in one position to no longer than 30 minutes. K.L. was also taught how to carry objects correctly.

Because the patient's muscles were completely loose and functioning well at this point in the therapeutic program, a closer evaluation of the skeletal condition was undertaken. This revealed that the lumbar curve did not have complete freedom of movement and the lumbar vertebrae lacked complete range of motion. Two exercises to increase the range of motion of the lumbar vertebrae were added to the program along with strenuous workouts on the Roman Chair.

On April 21, the patient reported that she had been able to increase her shopping, sitting, and working activities while remaining pain-free and was very happy with her present status. She requested and was given permission to swim while in California during the upcoming week, provided that the swim would be preceded by a good stretch.

Upon returning from the trip, K.L. was happy to report that she had been able to function well with only mild discomfort during the long periods of sitting. This discomfort had been alleviated by the utilization of the pain-relief methods taught during the educational aspect of the Body Techniques program.

Progress was noted at each successive treatment, and on May 7, the patient reported swimming ten laps with no ill effects. Her only complaint was mild soreness in the left hip and groin abductor region. In order to affect this area directly, an abdominal stretch on the Roman Chair was given following the usual treatment protocol of modality application, Body Techniques, and exercise review. It was obvious that the patient was feeling better because for the first time she was interested in losing weight and improving her appearance. Her total mind-set was not toward getting better but on looking as healthy as she felt.

Because the therapist realized that Patient K.L. was not yet ready for the strain of the Sit Up/Sit Back exercise, two abdominal exercises were added to gently strengthen the patient's abdominals. These were lift ups (not curl ups) to the side for the oblique abdominal muscles and in the straight plane for the rectus abdominis. They were to be performed supine with knees bent, while lifting the upper body as a unit *without* bending in the thoracic area or bringing the head forward. These exercises are preliminary to the more strenuous Sit Up/Sit Back.

Treatments continued with each session consisting of modality application, exercise review, condition reassessment, and introduction of progressive exercises to continue Ms. K.L. in the Corrective Phase of her therapy. At this stage the modalities were pulsed Ultrasound, Medcolator, heat to the left low back, and electrical stimulation to the left buttock and left hip abductor. Exercises were also being specifically directed to these areas. The patient had progressed to swimming 18 laps a day in conjunction with an extensive exercise program with no ill effects.

On June 11, treatment included a prone Hip Extension exercise for the gluteus maximus and hamstring muscles with a five pound weight in both fast and slow components and a PRE for the left hip abductor.

On July 19, the patient related that she was able to tolerate rock climbing, gardening, and swimming during the past weekend, with absolutely no back pain. She did complain of some stiffness which was normal for such a vigorous increase in activity.

On August 9, K.L. returned to treatment after an extended absence caused by traveling. She was and had been pain-free except for the left rectus femoris which had cramped during long periods of sitting, especially during the flight. The therapist introduced several rectus femoris stretches and advised the patient to direct the bulk of her home exercise program to a concentration in that area.

On September 9, a periodic reevaluation indicated that the patient was pain-free and her remaining problems were in the functional area. Ms. K.L. was under the impression that she could work 16 stress-filled hours a day, swim an hour, and practice yoga for one-half hour without her body rebelling. It became the therapist's goal, during extensive dialogue, to attempt to establish realistic expectations for physical activity within the structure of this patient's demanding lifestyle. In K.L.'s case, these realistic activity goals translated into swimming two to three times a week, mild yoga and relaxation one time a week, Body Techniques treatment once every second week, and a Roman Chair workout two times a week in addition to the treatment sessions. She was also advised to begin Nautilus at the local Y.M.C.A. to increase total body strength.

Subjectively, during this reevaluation, K.L. reported feeling much better and healthier. She had an occasional problem with sitting for long periods of time, in certain positions, and when bending/twisting to the left. She was now able among other things to swim three to four times a week and practice yoga. Because she was still not as active as she desired, the therapist added three new exercises at this time: another Hip Flexor Stretch using a chair; a Standing Groin Stretch with rotation to get to the rotators of the left hip; and the straight back Sit Up/Sit Back which the patient was finally able to execute.

After almost a full year of treatment, K.L. was at the point where she needed guidance in returning to a more natural lifestyle where she could still accomplish her ambitious goals but also have an exercise program that would both relieve her stress and keep her musculo-skeletal systems balanced. If she lived a life which was much less demanding on her physically and emotionally, her rehabilitation would have been accomplished in a shorter period of time. Because she insisted upon placing such tremendous demands on her body she would often times negate some of the productive work done during treatment by overdoing normal daily living activity. At this point, when her body did rebel, a treatment of Body Techniques relieved the symptoms. She was also able to relieve any pain or stressful symptoms through execution of her exercise program.

A unique aspect of this case surfaced in October, when K.L. announced that she was pregnant. Modalities and Body Techniques were immediately changed to accommodate her new condition, and the therapist reassured the patient that the pregnancy should not destroy the gains made over the last year. However, it was decided (by the therapist in conjunction with the obstetrician) that rather than a discharge it would be wise to continue therapeutic sessions periodically in order to prevent any exacerbation of pain.

Summary

This case illustrates many important facets of the Body Techniques treatment program. It exhibits the change in modalities as the patient's condition changes; the constant examination of the patient; the change in treatment protocol based on the reassessments; the education of the patient at all times; and the gearing of the program to the patient's lifestyle needs with advice on how to carry this information into everyday health maintenance.

Case History #5—Tennis Elbow and Cervical Radiculopathy on the Right Side

Mr. P.L. was referred by a physician for the treatment of tennis elbow. During the Initial Evaluation two separate but related problems were noted, i.e., tennis elbow on the right and a previous medical history of a cervical radiculopathy on the right. The physician did not think that there was a relationship between the two conditions.

Initial Evaluation

- Triggerpoints and muscle spasms in the right cervical muscles
- Triggerpoints at the right medial border of the scapula
- Decreased range of motion in the right supinator; right shoulder complex; scapula; cervical joints; and especially in right shoulder flexion
- Poor posture with the forward head position
- Trunk weakness
- Negative X-rays

Treatment Goals

- Decrease muscle spasms and triggerpoints
- Increase flexibility of all limited muscles

- Increase range of motion of all limited joints
- Increase the function of the cervical area, the shoulder girdle, the scapular area, and the right elbow

Patient P.L. received a total of 20 treatments and was discharged with full function, pain free, and able to play tennis without exacerbation. The initial treatment consisted of Ultrasound application and friction massage to the right wrist extensor tendon. During the application of Body Techniques in the sitting position, the therapist evaluated the right scapula and shoulder complex more deeply with palpation. In order to treat the cervical radiculopathy, it was necessary to first eliminate the symptomatic tennis elbow. This was accomplished by the introduction of three tennis elbow exercises which were stretches for the wrist flexors, the extensors, and supinator. Ice was applied to the extensor tendon in addition to pulsed Ultrasound and alternating current.

The patient received several similar treatments for the tennis elbow until the pain was eliminated during normal functional activity. In conjunction with the exercise program that the patient was performing (to treat the tennis elbow) the therapist was working on the cervical and scapular areas on the right side. The Body Techniques program, consisting of ice/heat, Ultrasound, and electrotherapy modalities combined with Body Techniques manipulation, and Body Movements, was followed in the treatment of the radiculopathy.

Several exercises were added to Patient P.L.'s program in order to increase the range of motion of the scapula. The Scapula Pull, in which the patient places his arms across his chest and tries to reach the left scapula with his right hand and the right scapula with the left hand as he bends over and breathes, was one of these manual stretch exercises. The patient proceeds with the exercise until he can "pull" his scapulae forward. This particular exercise stretches the rhomboids and the middle trapezius and assists the patient in maintaining the increased range of motion of the scapulae which was reached during the treatment.

Patient P.L. continued with these tennis elbow and manual stretch exercises while adding new exercises to correct his posture and increase the range of motion in his limited joints. During the first five treatments, progress was noted in the treatment of the tennis elbow but not in the neck or scapula. During the 6th treatment, a greater range of motion was discovered in the neck, the spasms were released, and the patient had gained complete pain-free mobility of his arm. From that time on, the range of motion in the cervical area began progressing and improving rapidly. Specific mobilization of the right scapula was accomplished along with Body Techniques at this treatment session.

The major restriction noted during the 8th treatment session was in the right trapezius from the mid-occiput attachment to the AC joint.

Therefore, the modalities were changed to concentrate on this area with Ultrasound applications to this muscle and its attachments to help achieve the desired flexibility. This was followed by heat, Medcolator, and vigorous stretching. The patient continued to improve at a rapid rate. A reevaluation of the condition of Mr. P.L. at this time indicated that he was able to hold his posture better; there was no tennis elbow pain; there was increased range of motion of the neck; the scapula was loosening up; there was no pain in that area; and the only restrictions to regaining good head position were the right trapezius muscle and a remaining lack of full scapula range of motion. These two areas became the concentration areas for successive treatment sessions.

During the 16th treatment, the patient reported that he had played tennis several times with no pain in the elbow. The final four treatment sessions concentrated upon continued stretching of the trapezius, Body Techniques to define any deep underlying areas of spasm or trigger-points, and modalities applications to areas of need. Although the patient was placed under intense stress at work during this time in his treatment plan, there was no exacerbation of pain in the cervical area. Patient P.L. was discharged at the end of his 20th treatment completely pain-free, with normal range of motion in all affected joints, proper body posture, and an increase in functional and recreational activities.

Summary

This middle-aged patient presented with two serious medical problems, i.e., cervical radiculopathy and a painful tennis elbow, which was limiting both his normal functional and recreational activities. It is much more difficult to treat a cervical radiculopathy in older patients because of old habits and the degeneration which naturally occurs in people of advanced years.

Body Techniques was the vital aspect in treating these two medical conditions by evaluating the existing dysfunctions correctly; eliminating the triggerpoints; reducing the spasms; loosening the tight muscles; stretching the restrictive muscles; and specifically mobilizing the scapula. The range of motion exercises for the neck and the scapula, education in postural awareness, Body Movements, and therapeutic exercise taught the patient how to maintain the correct posture after it was regained. Patient P.L. was able to return to his normal daily and recreational activities with no pain or restriction.

Case History #6—Emergency Treatment for Acute Muscle Spasm and Lumbar Radiculopathy on the Left Side

Patient P.H. received an emergency treatment for extreme pain in the low back which traveled to the left lateral thigh, left groin, and the left knee. The pain had begun four days prior to treatment as Mr. P.H., who is 72 years of age, was getting out of a golf cart. There was an increase in pain upon weight bearing. Previous treatment had included diagnostic x-rays which were negative, hot soaks, and analgesics without relief. The Initial Evaluation was incomplete because of the intensity of the pain, therefore the initial treatment consisted of Medcolator application (five minutes tetanizing—fifteen minutes surge) to the muscle spasm in the left quadriceps (four pads) and left and right low back, with a 15-minute surge application to the left and right gluteal muscles. Ice was applied to the low back and the patient was also instructed in Deep Breathing, Head Wobble, and Knee to Chest Body Movements. Body Techniques was also performed on the patient in the prone and supine positions. The second treatment consisted of the same modalities with the addition of hip rolling to assist in breaking the spasm patterns.

Because the patient's pain was under control, treatment 3 began with a continuation of the previously incomplete Initial Evaluation and elicited the following information:

- Original pain was reproduced by hip flexion of the left hip
- Forward flexion: 9½ inches from the floor
- Hamstrings: left 70 degrees; right 52 degrees
- Tightness: extreme in left rectus femoris and left adductor; moderate in right hip flexor
- Triggerpoints: left occiput, left buttocks, left inferior angle of the scapula
- Weakness: left hamstring, left abductor, right adductor
- Standing Side-Bend: left side extremely tight

Impression

This patient had extremely restricted musculature around the left hip. His lumbar vertebrae were immobile, and his trunk musculature had been severely weakened by the constant wearing of a girdle to relieve occasional back pain. The patient also had an extreme forward head position with protracted shoulders.

Treatment Goals

- Eliminate functional pain
- Increase flexibility of the muscles of the left hip and the low back
- Mobilization of the lumbar vertebrae through exercise (because of patient's age)
- Strengthening of weakened muscles
- Regain normal range of motion in limited joints
- Improvement of total body posture

Treatment Plan

- Continuation of previous modality applications plus pulsed Ultra-sound to the triggerpoints as listed
- Active and passive stretching around the pelvis
- Corrective exercises to include: introduction of the Knee Drop with Breathing to begin to get range of motion of the lumbar vertebrae; hip extension on three pillows; stretching of piriformis, hip flexors, and rectus femoris bilaterally
- PREs to weakened muscles
- Continuation of Body Techniques and therapeutic exercises

Summary

Patient P.H. was discharged after the 13th treatment at which time he was pain-free with occasional twinges in the low back. He was pleased with his progress and did not feel that he would be diligent in performing any further exercises. With a patient this advanced in years and with such a small degree of motivation, the standard program of strengthening was replaced by a few gentle exercises for the trunk which would work the abdominal and buttock muscles.

Body Techniques accomplished improved posture and an increased range of motion in the neck, shoulders, back, and pelvic areas. Even though this patient's age was a factor in the prognosis for recovery, the flexibility of Body Techniques allowed a complete cure to be attained in a short period of time.

Case History #7—Severe Lumbar Radiculopathy with Sciatica

Patient M.K. is a woman in her 30s who had delivered a baby four months previous to her initial consultation. She exhibited postpartum back pain which made walking almost impossible. Because of the severity of the symptoms, the weakness of her abdominal muscles which had not rebounded from the strain of pregnancy, and the necessity of continual exposure to the repeated stress (lifting the infant) which had caused the back pain originally, a thermomold corset was prescribed to replace the abdominal muscles which were absent at this time.

Initial Evaluation

Symptomatology:
- Severe radiation of pain to the left side, left buttock, and left leg
- Pain increased with urination and defecation
- Unable to stand, sit, or walk for any length of time
- Problem aggravated by carrying and lifting her child

Structural Abnormalities:
- Forward head position and thoracic slump with history of severe headaches
- Pelvis was increased on the left
- Right shoulder was increased
- Patient was 5 inches from the floor in forward flexion
- Muscle spasm in the right trapezius

Weakness:
- Left hip adductor
- Left hip abductor
- Left hamstring
- Trunk in general

Flexibility:
- Hamstrings: right = 85 degrees; left = 55 degrees
- Extreme tightness in the left rectus femoris which elicited an exacerbation of the original pain

Treatment Goals

- Decrease pain
- Improve posture
- Stretch restricted muscles
- Strengthen weak muscles
- Return patient to full, pain free, functional lifestyle

This patient's initial treatments consisted of cryotherapy, Medcolator applications, and prone and supine Body Techniques. She received information on proper ice applications for home use and was instructed to hold in her abdominals. Because of the severity of the pain, it was impossible to introduce any further exercises for the abdominals at this time. The Body Movements were introduced with special care being taken with the Hip Extension on Pillows. This was to be executed gently until the patient just began to feel the pain at which point she was to stop the exercise. The goal of the Hip Extension exercise was to *gain the benefit of the exercise without an exacerbation of the pain.*

The patient gradually improved and during the 4th treatment reported freedom from pain unless induced by carrying the baby on a hip, standing for a long time, or bending without the brace. The Cat Back exercise was executed at this time without pain exacerbation.

M.K. reported at the next appointment that the back pain had returned without an increase or change in activity level. Upon extensive questioning it was deduced that she was nursing the baby in a very awkward position. Instruction was given in a method of back protection while engaging in this activity and the back pain disappeared.

Therapy progressed to include the Standing Side-Bend and an exercise to stretch out the protracted shoulders. At this point work was being done on strengthening the abdominals without straining the back and correcting the patient's posture in order to relieve the negative mechanical forces of unequal weight distribution, which would continue to exacerbate the radiculopathy if not corrected at this time.

When the Hip Flexor Stretch was added to the program it was very painful and required a great deal of instruction in proper execution while breathing through the pain. However, once M.K. mastered the technique, the patient received so much relief that a great deal of effort was put into the exercise and extensive benefit was therefore gained from it.

Strengthening exercises were added for the left hip abductor, the left hamstring, and the left adductor with a five pound cuff weight. Three treatments later (a total of 25 treatments), this patient was discharged totally pain-free and has remained in this condition throughout a year of active motherhood.

Summary

Patient M.K. expressed the manifestation of the additional benefit of stress and tension relief during the Body Techniques and home exercise program. Since this patient's focus was on a total holistic health plan (homeopathic care, vegetarian diet, and medicinal herb therapy from other sources) the drug-free, self-healing, patient-controlled aspects of the Body Techniques program and the rapidity of the cure fit nicely into her lifestyle.

Case History #8—Arachnoiditis, Radiculopathy, Bilateral Sciatica (Postlaminectomy, Fusion, Implant)

Every health practitioner must face the fact that regardless of the efficacy of the particular treatment being applied, there are patients who will not respond positively to the care being given. The therapist can often conclude during the Initial Evaluation that a certain patient exhibits attitudes which will be counter-productive. The decision must then be made as to the wisdom of refusing treatment to this particular patient knowing that the therapy will most likely be ineffective because of the patient's past proclivity to failure. Because the Body Techniques program is so flexible and includes the patient's psychological profile in the total planning of the treatment protocol, it would seem in all fairness to the patient that the treatment should be attempted until there is absolute proof that the therapist's original judgment was correct. In the case of Patient A.H., the previous medical history indicated a psychological overlay which would more than likely preclude effective treatment.

Initial Evaluation

Medical History: Mr. A.H. is a frail, deconditioned man of 60 who had received a laminectomy, spinal fusion, two rhizotomies, numerous drug therapies, and finally the insertion and subsequent removal of a spinal stimulator for pain control. During removal of the electrical implant, a wire was left in the soft tissue of the back, and the patient refused further surgery for removal.

Patient Profile: This patient presented with debilitating weakness, extensive scarring of the left low back, and a residual three-inch wire in the lower left side. He was severely stooped, listed to one side, and exhibited depression and intense negativity. He was presently receiving psychiatric and neurological care with drug therapy and had been referred to physical therapy by the attending physician.

It was impossible to complete an Initial Evaluation on this patient due to the severity of pain and the debilitation of his overall condition, therefore after consultation with his surgeon and neurologist, therapy was initiated for pain relief. It should be noted here that previous X-rays, myelograms, and CAT scans were negative and that Mr. A.H. tested out as being 17 inches from the floor in forward flexion. He exhibited poor posture with forward head position and thoracic kyphosis.

Treatment Goal

The goal was to alter the perception of, and reaction to, pain. Because of the mental and physical condition of the patient, it was obvious that the pain would not be relieved easily. It was therefore necessary to change his conception of pain before it ever would be possible to reduce his reaction to pain.

Treatment Plan

Patient A.H. was treated with Medcolator and ice to the low back and buttocks bilaterally. Body Techniques were applied very lightly because of the fraility of the patient. The therapist had to assist Mr. A.H. in each movement on the plinthe. During his successive treatments, instruction was given in correct breathing techniques, the Head Wobble, Neck Push, Knees to Chest, and Pelvic Tilt with Neck Push. An area of muscle spasm was discovered at the right iliac crest and was treated with Ultrasound. Much to the disapproval of the patient, a Bend/Sit exercise was attempted with the assistance of the therapist. He had been advised many times before by various practitioners "never" to bend his back, which made normal movement impossible. Further treatment sessions included, along with the modalities, introduction of the Side/Stretch while standing, buttocks pinches between each exercise, and the Cat Back with supervision.

Treatment Progression

On the surface, Mr. A.H. was being cooperative and positive about the therapy. Because of a desire to prove to all concerned that every available treatment was being tried for the alleviation of his condition, this patient indicated a willingness to participate actively in the therapeutic program. Upon investigation, however, it became apparent that he was only verbalizing his cooperation. The home exercise program was not being executed because the patient claimed it intensified his pain and, because he did not like the ice, would not reduce the pain through cryotherapy.

Office treatment sessions were invariably interfered with by numerous complaints of other physical problems such as intestinal discomfort. Every time the therapist would begin to apply the Body Techniques, a source of discomfort unrelated to the back would arise which would cause a lessening of the treatment or a discontinuation of a certain phase of the plan for that session. In other words, Patient A.H. was continually undermining the program while professing to be totally cooperative.

Another aspect of this case which should be recognized is the support group manipulation. At each session Mr. A.H. was attended by at least two family members who catered to him and whose lives revolved around the pain of their loved one. It was obvious that the family was being kept under control by the pain and health needs of this patient.

Psychological therapy based upon the reinforcement by the therapist of only positive movements and attitudes, when found, was ineffective. A tough approach, in an attempt to bully A.H. into cooperating in his own health care, also did not work. Every avenue of approach attempted in the Body Techniques psychological area was to no avail because Mr. A.H., himself, had not yet decided that he was ready to "get better." He continued to maintain complete control of his pain. It was also difficult to teach any of the exercise program because previous health care practitioners had instructed the patient not to bend his back to any degree, and each movement met with resistance. Every time discomfort was felt it was verbally interpreted by the patient as debilitating pain and thus precluded any further movement in that area.

Body Techniques therapy was continued under these inhibiting conditions for ten sessions. At the end of these it was noted that Mr. A.H. had begun to make functional progress although he would not admit to either a degree of lessening of pain or to an increase in mobility. He was able to walk erectly, climb upon the plinthe unaided, and execute movements with a flexibility that had been previously impossible. He related that his neighbors had noticed the improvement in his ability to walk normally and had commented upon the obvious success of his therapeutic program. He would not admit to even a minute degree of progress, however.

The patient discontinued the therapy with a phone call informing the therapist that he was in such intense pain that he had contacted his neurologist and she had advised discontinuance of physical therapy and implemented increased drug therapy. Because of the signs of improvement which had begun to manifest themselves, regardless of Mr. A.H.'s negative mind-set, a phone consultation was sought by the therapist with the neurologist. However, the neurologist refused to cooperate with the therapist's wish to confront the patient in an attempt to force him to "give up" his pain. She merely mumbled that he needed a new psychiatrist and that she had prescribed a new drug for him. It was felt by the therapist that with the cooperation of the neurologist, the patient would be unable to further manipulate his health-care providers and would be forced to come to terms with the reality of the situation and hopefully a cure would then be possible. The neurologist disagreed and preferred increased drug therapy in conjunction with additional psychiatric treatment. It was unfortunate that the patient was able to continue to retain control over his family, friends, and environment by this manipulation of his primary care physician. He was now able to claim that he had tried everything to get better even though he had subtly not tried at all. It was quite revealing of this patient's true intent that as soon as the success of the therapy was pointed out by his increased performance level and by family and neighbors, an immediate avenue of escape was found. This poor, misguided individual actually ran from a program which would have enabled him to function within normal limits.

Summary

Body Techniques have the ability to induce functional changes even in the most uncooperative patient. In the final analysis, however, there is little possibility of cure in a patient who has made a science of manipulation and gains emotional need and satisfaction from continuation of his poor health.

Case History #9—Chest Pain

Patient H.J. is a middle-aged woman who had been experiencing chest pains which she feared were symptoms of a heart problem. Her physician assured her after all the appropriate testing that her heart was fine, but he had no answer for the source of pain. She was referred by a previously treated patient.

Initial Evaluation

- Extreme pain in the left shoulder area with radiation into the arm
- Movement of the left arm produced a stabbing chest pain of undetermined origin.
- Extreme and severe muscle spasm at the left medial border of the scapula

Treatment Plan

The initial treatment session included ice, Medcolator, and modified Body Techniques to release the muscle spasm and relieve the pain. The patient returned on the next day and was able to be further evaluated because the spasm had been broken and the pain had somewhat subsided. During this examination by palpation, a painful nodule was discovered on the left side of the vertebral column at approximately T1, 2, and 3 along with pain radiating from the costosternal joint at the same level at the sternum.

The goal of this particular treatment was to adjust the position of the rib cage. Therefore, the patient received modality and Body Techniques treatment plus mobilization of the joints of the sternum. The home program included gentle exercises to be performed at the doorway in order to increase the range of motion of the costosternal joints.

Patient H.J.'s treatment schedule continued with the application of gentle Body Techniques and mobilization of the scapula in the sitting position on the left. Pain was relieved in the sternum after eight sessions. The left scapula was the underlying cause of the dysfunction in this patient, therefore it received continual work. After 20 treatments the patient reported being at 90–95% efficiency in all functional activities. After two additional treatments she was discharged and has reported back on occasion that she is remaining active with complete freedom from restriction and pain.

Summary

This patient's problem was unable to be detected until the muscle spasm was broken and the therapist attempted to align the body. At that time, it was discovered that the rib cage was rotated. The therapist was able to duplicate the patient's pain and, therefore, was better able to identify the causal factor. Once the underlying dysfunction (the lack of range of motion of the left scapula that was putting abnormal pull on the rib cage during movement) was discovered, the therapy was concentrated on relieving that condition and realigning the patient's posture. She began to respond immediately to the treatment and quickly reached a pain-free and functionally healthy state.

Case History #10—Scoliosis/Spondylolisthesis

Patient K.I. is a young, female teacher who was referred by a physician from a large New York hospital. She used to be a very active person but at the time of her first visit was unable to walk a city block because of pain. A range of diagnostic testing, including a myelogram and CAT scan, had been ineffective in determining the cause of the pins and needles and numbness in her right leg which had begun one year ago. X-rays, however, identified a moderate spondylolisthesis at L5-S1 level. Due to the lifting, bending, and strenuous activity required in her position as a kindergarten teacher, from which she was unable to obtain a leave of absence, a thermomold corset was prescribed in order to counteract the stresses she encountered on a daily basis which were exacerbating the condition.

Initial Evaluation

- Overweight, poor posture, weak trunk muscles
- Pelvis elevated on left ½ inch
- 8 inches from floor in forward flexion
- No movement in lumbar or thoracic vertebrae
- Hamstrings: right = 63 degrees; left = 85 degrees
- Muscle testing of right hamstring, abductor, and hip flexor caused exacerbation of pain
- Right side bend indicated tightness
- Increased lumbar lordosis
- Forward head position
- Scoliosis
- Muscle spasm in low back

Impression

Patient has poor posture due to: scoliosis, muscle imbalance, structural abnormalities, and incapacitating pain.

Treatment Goal

- To relax all muscles and regain muscular balance
- To reduce the mechanical effects of scoliosis and spondylolisthesis as much as possible
- To decrease excessive forward head position
- To correct general posture

Treatment Plan

K.I. had a total of 15 treatments consisting of heat/cold, Ultrasound, Medcolator, Body Techniques, therapeutic exercise, and postural alignment. Because this patient lived a considerable distance from the treatment center, as soon as she was relatively pain-free a transfer to a therapist closer to her home was arranged. A follow-up phone call revealed that K.I. had ceased exercising, failed to continue the physical therapy treatments, and had returned to the care of a neurologist who had decided to prescribe further diagnostic testing and finally surgery because of the reappearance of the symptomatology.

Summary

Body Techniques can make a difference with a structural problem in the skeletal system such as spondylolisthesis and/or scoliosis. However, with structural abnormalities it is even more important than usual for the patient to carry out his part of the program by continuing on the daily prescribed exercise regimen to remove as many negative mechanical forces as possible. The Body Techniques program accomplishes this goal by correcting any restrictions, aligning the skeletal system, and strengthening weak muscles so they will hold the corrected position by teaching the patient to maintain the correct posture during functional activity. This patient received the benefits of the program as exhibited by her pain-free state (minus the corset) after 15 treatments. However, when she discontinued the home treatment regimen, the symptoms returned.

Case History #11—Cervical Dysfunction/ Lumbar Radiculopathy

Patient F.D. presented with a complicated medical history which included lumbar laminectomy (two levels), spinal fusion, and lumbar stenosis. At the present time, a cervical dysfunction was causing severe neck pain and exacerbating her back pain which was in turn interfering with her functional activities. Previous surgery and non-aggressive physical therapy had proved ineffective and she had been left in a back brace which she felt was further complicating her condition. Needless to say, Ms. F.D. was both frustrated and bewildered as to the best course to follow when she arrived at our office. The following is her initial musculo-skeletal profile.

Initial Evaluation:

Skeletal:
- forward head position with limitation at atlanto-occipital joint
- lack of mobility in lower thoracic/lumbar area (partly due to fusion)
- pelvic obliquity, increased on left
- increased height of left shoulder

Muscular:
- severe muscle spasms in cervical and scapular areas
- triggerpoints at occiput bilaterally (increased on left) and medial border of scapula
- extremely weak muscles, especially low back/abdominals

Functional:
- patient wears a lumbo-sacral brace constantly
- chronically weak trunk musculature has caused a forward-head, thoracic-slumped posture

Treatment of patient F.D. consisted of Body Techniques, reassurance, program explanation, postural alignment, and balancing of the muscular system. Ms. F.D. is very tall and this, in conjunction with her complicated medical history, caused difficulty in the achievement of correct posture. The Treatment of Pain and Corrective Phases of her program extended over an eight month period of time and were effective. She is presently in the Preventive Phase where she is receiving a weekly treatment whose chief goals are to strengthen weak trunk muscles and correct the improper head position. These two areas of concern are the only remaining problems for this patient as she is relatively pain-free, able to function normally without the use of the brace, leads a very active life, and has surprised her physician with her recovery.

Ms. F.D. is not a person who exercises well or independently, and therefore the weekly therapeutic session not only strengthens weak areas but also provides the therapist with an opportunity to follow her progress, motivate her, encourage her, and continue to align her posture.

Summary

Body Techniques was used in this case for postsurgical rehabilitation and postural alignment. The Treatment of Pain Phase alleviated the muscle spasms and triggerpoints while the Corrective Phase increased mobility in the thoracic/lumbar areas as well as balancing the pelvis and shoulders. The patient's postural problems will continue to be treated in the Preventive Phase. The physical success and the attendance to the patient's psychological needs changed Ms. F.D. from frustrated and confused to hopeful and directed. Treatment protocol utilized each and every aspect of the Body Techniques program to effect a successful return of this patient to a full and satisfying lifestyle.

Case History #12—Scoliosis/Whiplash

Ms. H.N. was referred by her attending physician for treatment of traumatic myositis resulting from a motor vehicle accident which had taken place six months previously. Prior treatment had consisted of chiropractics and orthopedics, neither of which had lastingly affected her condition. At this time she was unable to participate in regular activities because the pain restricted her to short periods of sitting, walking, or driving.

Initial Evaluation

- Pain in the cervical area, mid-back, and low back
- Stiffness in cervical joints
- Muscle spasm of left trapezius muscle along entire right paraspinal muscle
- Triggerpoints at left occiput, left iliac crest
- Locked, immobile OA joint on left
- Forward head position due to muscular pain and limitation
- General posture poor and reinforcing cervical, mid-back, and low-back pain

Patient was treated with cryotherapy, electrotherapy, Body Techniques, postural alignment, and therapeutic exercises to correct these deficiencies. Her program was progressing well for two months when she sustained an exacerbation of the muscle spasm due to a second motor vehicle accident. Treatment of the muscle spasm was added to the primary corrective therapy in operation at that time. She was discharged pain-free and functional three months after initial consultation.

Summary

The recurrence of muscle spasm caused by the second trauma placed H.N. concurrently in two Phases of the Body Techniques program. The ability of Body Techniques to treat several areas of need simultaneously allows the therapist the flexibility of management which is essential for a continuously successful rehabilitation program.

Summary

Both the flexibility and the structure of Body Techniques is demonstrated by the case history presentations. The individual care and consideration given to each patient is as vital as the level of the practitioner's professional judgment and skill. With practice, dedication, and patience, the health practitioner of today will find Body Techniques to be a complete and useful therapeutic approach with which he or she can effectively become a catalyst and supporter of the patient's healing process in a humane and safe manner.

BIBLIOGRAPHY

Barlow, W. (1973). *The Alexander Technique.* Alfred A. Knopf, New York.

Basmajian, J. V. (1978). *Therapeutic Exercise.* Williams & Wilkins, Baltimore.

Benson, H. (1979). *The Mind/Body Effect.* Simon & Schuster, New York. Paperback ed.: Berkley Books, New York (1980).

Brown, J. H. U. (1979). *The Health Care Dilemma.* Human Sciences Press, New York.

Burke, R. E. (1978). Motor Units: Physiological/Histochemical Profiles, Neural Connectivity and Functional Specializations. *Am. Zool.,* 18:127–134.

Costa, E., and Greengard, P. (Eds). (1979). Brain peptides: A new endocrinology. In *Advances in Biochemical Psycho-pharmacology, Vol. 20.* Raven Press, New York.

Collu, R. et al. (Eds.) *Central Nervous System Effects of Hypothalamic Hormones and Other Peptides.* Raven Press, New York, pp. 237–301.

Cyriax, J. (1975). *Textbook of Orthopaedic Medicine. Diagnosis of Soft Tissue Lesions. Vol. 1.* 6th ed. Bailliere Tindall, Williams & Wilkins, Baltimore, Maryland.

Cyriax, J., and Russell, G. (1977). *Textbook of Orthopaedic Medicine. Vol. 2.* 9th ed. Bailliere Tindall, London.

Kraus, H. (1970). *Clinical Treatment of Back and Neck Pain.* McGraw Hill, New York.

Fisk, J. W., et al. (1977). *The Painful Neck and Back, A Practical Guide to Management of Diagnosis, Manipulation, Exercises, Prevention.* Charles C Thomas, Springfield, Ill.

Vrbova, G., Gordon, T., Jones, R. (1980). *Nerve-Muscle Interaction.* Chapman and Hall, London. A Halsted Press Book. John Wiley & Sons, New York.

Goldstein, M. (Ed.). (Feb. 1975) *The Research Status of Spinal Manipulative Therapy.* U.S. Dept. of Health, Education and Welfare, Public Health Service, National Institute of Health. NINCDS Monograph. No. 15. Workshop at Bethesda. Maryland. DHEW Publication No. (NIH) 76-998.

Guillemin, R. (1979). Current studies on beta-endorphins and enkephalins. In *Brain Peptides: A New Endocrinology* A. M. Gotto, Jr., E. J. Peck Jr., A. E. Boyd III (Eds.). Elsevier North Holland Biomedical Press.

Guyton, A. C. (1981). *Medical Physiology* 6th ed. W.B. Saunders Co., Philadelphia, London, Toronto.

Hosobuchi (1979) *Science* 203, in above study edited by Gotto, etc.

Ingber, D. (June 1981). Brain Breathing. *Science Digest.*

Jackson, R. (1978). *The Cervical Syndrome.* Charles C Thomas. Springfield, Illinois.

Jones, R. T. (5/7/66). Vascular Changes Occurring in the Cervical Musculoskeletal System. *South Afr Med J.*

Kelsey, J. L., Pastides, H., Bisbee, G. E. Jr. (1978). Musculoskeletal disorders: Their frequency of occurrence and their impact on the population of the United States. *Prodist.* New York.

Krieger, D. (1979). *The Therapeutic Touch.* Prentice-Hall, Englewood Cliffs, New Jersey.

Lee, J. M., Warren, M. P., Mason, S. M. (1978). Effects of Ice of Nerve Conduction Velocity. *Physiotherapy.* Vol. 64, no. 1.

Lomax, E. (1975). Manipulative therapy: An historical perspective. In *Approaches to the Validation of Manipulation Therapy.* Charles C Thomas, Springfield, Ill. Proceedings of the International Congress on Approaches to the Validation of Manipulation Therapy.

Maitland, G. D. (1980). *Peripheral Manipulation.* Butterworth & Co. Ltd., London, Boston, Sydney, Toronto.

Masters, R. Houston, J. (1978). *Listening to the Body.* Dell, New York.

Moll, J., Wright, V. (1978). *Measurement of Spinal Movement in The Lumbar Spine and Back Pain.*

New England Journal of Medicine 1981; 304:638–42.

The New Physician March 1979 p. 55.

Oyle, I. (1979).*The New American Medicine Show.* Unity Pres, Santa Cruz, California.

Payton, Hirt, and Newton (1977). *Scientific Bases for Neurophysiologic Approaches to Therapeutic Exercise. An Anthology.* F. A. Davis Co., Philadelphia.

Rosse, C., Clawson, D. K. (1980). *The Musculoskeletal System in Health and Disease.* Harper & Row, Hagerstown, Md.

Shriber, W. J. (1975). *A Manual of Electrotherapy.* 4th ed. Lea & Febiger, Philadelphia.

Simmons, D. J., Kunn, A. S. (Eds.). (1979). *Skeletal Research: An Experimental Approach.* Academic Press, New York.

Simon, W. H. (Ed.). (1978). *The Human Joint in Health and Disease.* "Abnormal Joint Biomechanics" Wilson C. Hayes. University of Penn. Press.

Shannahoff-Khalsa, D. (1/3/83). *Brain-Mind Bulletin,* Salk Institute for Biological Studies.

Stoddard, A. (1980). *Manual of Osteopathic Techniques.* Hutchinson, London.

Usdin, E., Bunney, W. E., Jr., Kline, N. S. (Eds.). (1979). *Endorphins in Mental Health Research.* Oxford University Press, New York.

Wyke, B. D. (1979). Neurological mechanisms in the experience of pain. *Acupuncture and Electrotherapy. Research.* 4: 27.

        (1981). Neuro-K: Overcoming Disability with Sensory Awareness Training. *Brain/ Mind Bulletin.*

Youcha, G. (June 1981). Psychiatrists and folk magic. *Science Digest.*

Index